I0450717

Strength Training
for Women Only

Strength Training
for Women Only

How to Double Your Strength
in Only Six Weeks!

Joseph F Mullen

iUniverse, Inc.
New York Lincoln Shanghai

Strength Training for Women Only
How to Double Your Strength in Only Six Weeks!

All Rights Reserved © 2003 by Joseph F Mullen

No part of this book may be reproduced or transmitted in any form or by any means, graphic, electronic, or mechanical, including photocopying, recording, taping, or by any information storage retrieval system, without the written permission of the publisher.

iUniverse, Inc.
an imprint of iUniverse, Inc.

For information address:
iUniverse
2021 Pine Lake Road, Suite 100
Lincoln, NE 68512
www.iuniverse.com

Originally Published by:
Safe Life Journey Research Foundation
3rd Addition

ISBN: 0-595-28017-X

Printed in the United States of America

WARNING DISCLAIMER

This book is designed to provide information in regard to the subject matter covered. It is sold with the understanding that the publisher and author are not engaged in rendering legal, accounting or other professional services. If legal or other expert assistance is required, the services of a competent professional should be sought.

It is not the purpose of this book to reprint all the information that is otherwise available to the author and/or publisher; but to complement, amplify, copy and supplement other texts, You are urged to read all the available material, learn as much as possible about the subjects covered and to tailor the information to individual needs.

Every effort is made to make this manual as complete and accurate as possible, within the scope of the material. However, there may be mistakes both typographical and in content. Therefore, this text should be used only as a general guide and not as the ultimate source of physical therapy, medical billing, health and fitness and exercise information. Furthermore, this book contains information pertaining to the subjects discussed, only up to the printing date.

The purpose of this book is to educate and entertain. The author and Safe Life Journey Foundation, shall have neither liability nor responsibility to any person or entity concerning any loss or damage caused, or alleged to be caused, directly or indirectly by the information contained in this book.

If you do not wish to be bound by the above, you may return this book to the publisher for a refund.

In Just Six weeks, You Can Double Your Strength, Elevate Your Fitness Level and Improve Your Self-Esteem and Self-Reliance.

By Joseph Mullen

ACKNOWLEDGMENT

We have not attempted to cite in all text, all of the authorities and sources consulted in the preparation of our books. To do so requires more space than is available.

We sincerely thank everyone who has contributed, in person and through their knowledge sharing mediums, for contributing to the development of our publishing efforts and intellectual ammunition.

Especially, the early pioneers of high-tech exercise and Fitness Therapy. Their courage and research participation, allowed us to challenge the status quo and conduct research to benefit health and fitness professionals and ultimately consumers.

CONTENTS

FOREWORD

Fitness is fast becoming a way of life for a majority of the people. Historically, fitness is defined as "the absence of disease," and its attainment is associated with a physical training regimen involving exercise.

Presently, the definition of fitness, thanks to the Holistic Health movement, is encompassing not only the physical element, but is broadening to include all the known elements of wellness: the physical, mental, emotional, and spiritual essentials.

We believe a properly designed and supervised exercise program is the Gateway to total fitness and redefined as health or wellness. In this manual, we transcribe fitness to mean wellness.

Wellness by our definition means: The absence of any destructive disease, united with <u>above</u> average levels of strength, flexibility, muscular endurance, cardio respiratory endurance and <u>below</u> average levels of body fat.

When one experiences wellness, daily activities and on the job performance are easily performed, functional ability is maximal, sports performance is enhanced, and one has energy available for leisure activities.

Wellness provides greatly enhanced self-awareness, self-responsibility, and self-esteem. All of which are easily entered through the gateway of physical exercise.

Exercise itself will produce a certain level of wellness. One reaches a higher level of wellness when certain other components, related to the fitness environment, are controlled.

These components are as everything within the wellness environment identified by the five senses: sight, sound, smell, taste, and touch. Each of these is a principal contributor to the elevation of wellness or, if missing from the environment can contribute to the destruction of wellness.

We will outline how one can combine all of the requirements of wellness within a productive exercise program and within the exercise environment to produce maximum results in minimum time.

The potential for rapid wellness improvements is at the highest level it has ever been. Unfortunately, the manipulation of the consumer through the dissemination of misinformation, myths, superstitions and manipulation of the consumer has never been greater. Separating fact from fiction and truth from lies is a major objective of this manual.

The documented, independently researched knowledge within this manual is valid on all levels. It is free of the commercial or product bias usually found in the "fitness" industry.

Our recommendations will challenge the present perceptions of "proper" exercise. Our endeavor is to maintain a simple to understand, "how to" approach to the design and performance of a personal wellness program, and include important scientific information to the benefit of everyone.

We will share the highest levels of knowledge, backed by personal research, gained at the frontier of the fitness revolution.

It brings us much happiness to help you reach your goals quickly and safely.

Use this knowledge to your advantage.

YOU ARE UNIQUE

Yes, you are unique. Think of it! Millions live in the world and there is no one exactly like you, and if you are a twin, your brother or sister, will have certain characteristics different from yours.

A unique person faces choices that have a direct effect on your present and future lifestyle.
The choice you make regarding your wellness, appearance will determine how quickly, and safely you reach your wellness goals as related to an exercise program.

The right choices save you valuable time. Once wasted, time is gone forever. Many people forget that time is valuable when it applies to an exercise, and if one program does not work they will try another. More often than not, enthusiasm is lost. They become discouraged, retreat, and retire from exercise.

Others bounce from one program to another, like a pollinating bee buzzing from one flower to another. Instead they attempt every "quick weight loss diet" or the "latest fitness regimen" in spite of its apparent insanity.

The bee is on a clearly defined mission with a known purpose. It does not attempt to pollinate a stone or a tree stump. The bee recognizes its goal, limitations, and purpose. You must decide to clearly recognize yours.

Our purpose is to clearly define a dynamic, result producing wellness and exercise formula for you. We will help you see the role your Intent plays in your success, and tutor you in the significance of achieving success by allowing yourself permission to fail in a way that will not nullify your purpose.

You will learn how to accurately measure improvements on a daily basis and you will discover the time efficient, cost effective exercise system that guarantees results for everyone.

Any realistic goal you desire will be set into motion and becomes possible to achieve. You need not waste valuable time, become discouraged or injured.

All it takes is a sane, repeatable approach to exercise and weight management, and for you to embrace patience, perseverance, self discipline, and the spirit to believe you can do it and you will create it.

You can do it and we will guide you!

First, Determine Your Goal

Because you are unique, your dreams, visions, and goals are uniquely yours. Therefore, should your wellness program be unique and designed especially for you.

We mean designed for <u>all of you</u>: your physical, mental, emotional, and spiritual self. You are, after all, more than a physical self. Once you construct your exercise program, decide which tools to use, and accept the formulas in this book. When you do, all your elements will surface, improve, and transcend your non-visible physical, mental, emotional, and spiritual genetics.

For many years, intellectual plunder was committed on consumers by entrepreneurs who follow the old adage, stated: *"You will never go broke, underestimating the intelligence of the public."*

These charlatans continue to manipulate the emotions of trusting consumers in magazines, newspapers, on television radio and the World Wide Web. The cornucopia of useless knowledge and worthless products marketed by these thieves continue this pretension.

The result, many consumers are utterly confused about which information or products are legitimate. This book is an attempt set the record straight.

COMPARING YOU WITH OTHERS

It is realistic to feel some level of discouragement shortly after beginning an exercise program. This feeling is often based on assumptions that: (1) improvements are not happening fast enough or (2) others exercising in the same environment seems to work at a higher level than you do and her or his body responds quicker than mine.

These feelings are based in perceptions of one's view of exercise and self-consciousness around others in the exercise environment. The extra stress you place on yourself is countering productive to good health and obstructs progress. It is healthier to change one's perceptions.

All stress is self-imposed and can be self disposed. Start by reshaping your perceptions, and understanding the feelings are a natural by product of beginning a new lifestyle direction. Even with a good road map, it is easy to get lost. It is just as easy to get back on the road when you choose.

There is no rationally established data proving the kind of "average" improvements, you can expect at the beginning, middle, or end of an exercise program. There is only your average progress and it will differ from others.

Factors controlling progress are:

- Genetics.
- Intent.
- The design of your program.
- Exercise frequency.
- Recuperation time between exercise bouts.
- Nutrition.
- Weight management procedures.
- Stress level.
- Present level of self-esteem.
- Self-motivation.
- Self-responsibility.
- Commitment.

- Dedication.
- Living a balanced lifestyle.

It is vital to exercise at a level that you feel is appropriate for you. As you adjust to your new quest and the exercise environment, you will naturally increase the intensity of your workouts. We will talk about the work to rest period later in this manual.

There is no point continually beating you up about what you feel are "short comings". Usually, the short coming label you awarded yourself, is something you over rated, in comparison to how you feel about your own self worth in that special area. Do not deny your feelings because they are your feelings; however, you can place them in proper perspective. It is a certainty of life that it will change. Keep you eye on the prize and focus, focus, focus, on your goals. Do not get emotionally involved in self-criticism by falsely blaming yourself. Progress will not come on a moment-to-moment basic, or overnight, but they will come, and if you choose it to be, the developments will be permanent.

Compare yourself only to yourself; do not dwell on negativity or the past. Stay in present time and move forward!

ELEMENTAL TRUTH

The most common justifications for discouragement that contribute to the high exercise drop out rate are: (1) Fraudulent products, (2) Fitness memberships that never produce the promised results, (3) A misinformed personal knowledge base leading to unrealistic goal setting, (4) Fitness centers staffed by "instructor's" who fail to provide adequate supervision, education, and motivation.

Average physical fitness is defined as: The ability to live each day with vigor and alertness, without undue fatigue and pain, with energy left for leisure time activities.

Superior fitness will manifest itself by providing ABOVE average levels of strength, flexibility, muscular endurance, and cardio respiratory endurance. Another benefit of superior fitness is BELOW average levels of body fat.

Self-design of a wellness program requires a basic understanding of the requirements of productive fitness protocols to meet the goals you set for yourself.

It is not true that "something is better than nothing". Improperly planned exercise programs do more harm than good. Before launching a fitness program, check with your physician, and determine any restrictions he or she feel worth of your consideration. When in average health exercise is safe.

Although a fitness program can have profound, positive effects for your lifestyle, it may also cause serious damage to novice philosophies coupled with the too much—too soon attempt to hurry goals along.

There is no age barrier governing one's beginning of a fitness program. Attitude, not age is the major precondition, and everyone can benefit from exercise.

Men, women, and children can follow the same exercise program. Women will not develop "muscles like a man", children's physical growth will not be suppressed, and seniors can safely exercise when a common sense is exhibited.

A so-called average person can model the same program as an athlete. The only adaptation is in the relationship of the level of intensity to the person exercising.

"Intensity" by our definition represents the amount of time one rests between each set of exercise. The less rest allowed between exercises the higher the intensity. The more rest allowed the lower the intensity.

Those beginning an exercise program for the first time must gradually enter into high intensity exercise. Those formerly conditioned folks on a comeback quest should not attempt a high-intensity type program.

Proactive exercise can greatly reduce the chance of sports-related injuries, and will rehabilitate any injury incurred playing a favorite sport or simply stepping off a curbing. Common problems such as nagging lower back issues, knee, elbow, and shoulder injuries return to normal functional ability with sensible exercise.

Senior citizens, in particular, will benefit from safe exercise procedures. Bone thickness and body strength will increase, and aid in body balance and greater functional ability. Broken bones may be prevented as well experiencing improved mobility. Rising from a chair to a standing position, walking up and down stairs will become much easier.

In summary:

- Education is the key to understanding fitness training.
- Any realistic goal is achievable.
- Get your physician's OK.
- Most commonly accepted knowledge related to fitness is myth.
- Everyone will benefit from proper exercise.
- There are no age restrictions.
- Prevention and rehabilitation of injuries are possible.
- Permanent weight loss happens as one eats fewer calories than needed for daily activities.
- Strength, flexibility, muscular endurance, and cardio respiratory endurance are the foundations on which fitness is established.
- A properly designed wellness program will improve your physical, mental, emotional, and spiritual qualities. Spot reducing is a myth. Sauna wraps are useless and magic wands, lotions, potions, and pills do not exist.

Moreover, there is no tooth fairy.

Diet and Weight Management:
How to Lose Weight Quickly, Safely
And Permanently

"I eat like a bird, why do I gain weight" Whenever someone asks that question, and stares at me waiting for an answer, I ask "What kind of a bird, a sparrow or a vulture?"

Hundreds, perhaps thousands of books and millions of words focus on helping people lose weight. Some are fact based, many are fad based, and the books always place on the bestseller lists. Yet, people in America are fatter than ever. Does this seem like a contradiction to you?

Losing excess body weight is simple, if you follow certain systematic procedures; however, you cannot make up your own rules, or follow advice of the uniformed.

For instance, we once talked with the director of a woman's fitness center who was very misinformed. She believed the only way a woman who followed a weight training program, will not "develop muscles like a man," is to "Breathe out when lifting the weight."

Many-franchised diet plan consultants recommend that clients do no exercise of any type. Apparently, they do not know that if one diets without exercising, some of the body weight loss will be muscle tissue. Many medical journals agree.

Muscle tissue is "productive" tissue, and provides humans with the ability to so such things as sit, stand, and walk. It is important to retain as much muscle tissue as possible. If you exercise while dieting you will not lose muscle tissue.

Exercise and diet are two major components of weight loss. Two other major components to weight control are behavioral modification and a support system.

There are three elements to understand when determining how to go about weight management:

✓ If your body weight is staying about the same, you are in a state of <u>Caloric Balance</u>. Meaning: the amount of calories you are consuming is equal to the amount of calories you are using during your daily activities.

Daily activities include your thoughts, words, and actions throughout the day. For example, stress may not be a physical action, but it will affect the amount of calories one uses to get through the day.

✓ If your body weight increases slowly over a period: a week, a month, or yearly, you are in a state of <u>Positive Caloric Balance</u> and consuming more daily calories than you expend within daily activities.

If you notice that your weight decreases on a steady basis, you are in the state of Negative Caloric Intake and eating fewer calories than needed to complete daily activities.

Negative Caloric Intake is the condition one needs to remain in to lose body fat. Necessary daily energy comes from food intake, and is stored in the fat cells.

The weight loss takes place because the needed energy calories, when not eaten, are extracted from the body and used as the source of energy. In a sense, the fat converts to gasoline, burned and excreted from the body.

One little known phenomenon is that fat cells, although they shrink in size, never leave the body. If you decide to abandon your weight management program, and begin to enter into positive caloric intake, the fat cells expand and contain more fatty material than previously.

The result is that you will probably gain more body fat, and end up weighing more than before. This is very noticeable in those who are yo-yo dieters.

Just how does one decide how many calories are safe to eat and not gain weight? There are complex formulas used to arrive at the amount but we will use a simple formula. One we have used successfully with clients for decades.

All you need do is take your present body weight, and multiply it by the number 10 (if you are a sedentary person). If, as example, you weigh 150 pounds, multiply by 10 and the safe calorie amount is: 1500 calories.

If you are active, then use the multiple of 12 times your body's weight. If very active, use the multiple 15 to determine you daily caloric allowance.

This is a guesstimate, but an excellent starting point. The total calories may be increased or reduced later, but for now 1500 calories are safe amounts for a person weighing 150 pounds. Consult with your physician if you doubt this figure.

Total calorie intake is vital to weight loss, and you must determine how to distribute them in proportions of protein, carbohydrate, and fat.

This approach has many different recommendations from many different practitioners. What we are about to share with you is not written in stone, but has worked with many, many people who had no medical problems.

Years ago, we hired a Professor of Nutrition from a prestigious New England to construct basic food plans for our clientele. We used these guidelines for many years with great success. We share these with you for use only after checking with your physician.

These food plans were typically high in carbohydrate calories (65%), medium in protein calories (20%), and low in fat calories (15%).

In recent years, we interchanged that balance and now advise a mix of 40% carbohydrate, 30% protein, and 30% fat. These are the amounts recommended by the popular *Zone* books written by Barry Sears. For detailed information on this approach, we recommend you refer to his books.

Let us move forward assuming you will choose a plan that meets your physical, mental, emotional, and spiritual needs.

Having chosen the total amount of calories allowed, and decided on the mix of calories you will use, there is one more item to decide. How many meals a day should you eat?

More weight disappears when you eat several small meals a day rather than three large meals. In practice, this means to divide the 1500 calories into six or seven meals.

First meal is breakfast; second meal in between breakfast and lunch; next meal is lunch; next is a meal between lunch and dinner; then dinner and a final small meal about one hour before bed.

As you do this, the first development you notice is a major upswing in your energy level; then you will seldom be hungry. The munches will be a thing of the past. Does this sound intriguing?

One work of warning: There will be a 10 day to 14 day "lag time" related to weight loss. Once you begin your diet, do not expect to see any significant weight loss for at least 10 days, and up to 14 days.

It takes the body's metabolic system a time to adjust to a reduction in food intake. Imagine eating 3,500 calories and reducing your intake to 1,500 calories.

The first reaction of your metabolic system is that it believes you are in a caloric trauma. It reacts as if you are not eating enough fuel to support your basic metabolic needs, and provide energy for your daily activities. It decides to hold on to its fuel reserves, meaning: the body fat you have already accumulated.

Before starting your weight management program, your metabolic thermostat was set to burn calories at a certain amount per minute. Decreasing your fuel supplies causes the metabolic thermostat to slow the amount of calories it would typically use during the day.

The time for the metabolic system to feel you are not starving to death, and all is safe, is 10 to 14 days. Then, the thermostat resets to burn more calories per minute than it did previously.

At that point, you will begin to use body fat at the rate of 1 to 3 pounds per week. The amount of fat you lose is based on your caloric intake and you daily activity level.

At no time should you eat less than 1,000 calories per day without being under the care of a physician.

Many people assume that if X amount of calories will help them lose weight, eating fewer calories will cause faster weight loss. This is not true.

What happens is that your metabolic furnace will not reset itself from the trauma of lower caloric intake and fat loss slows to a trickle.

Stick with the formula of using your present body weight and multiplying it by 10 to decide how many calories to eat on a daily basis. If, at a point your weight loss levels off, increase your activity level to continue the loss. Always check with your physician before drastically reducing your caloric intake.

Along with a reduction in calories and an increase in activity levels, your diet should also:

- ✓ Satisfy all nutrient needs.
- ✓ Be acceptable to meet individual tastes and habits, including religious standards.
- ✓ Minimize hunger and fatigue.
- ✓ Be readily available and socially acceptable.
- ✓ Favor establishment of a lasting pattern of eating.
- ✓ Be conducive to improvement of overall health.

We have covered the basic dietary information related to safe, effective weight loss. Now, let us outline some behavioral modification and support suggestions.

Behavior modification is the most difficult weight loss component to master. Space does not allow an in-depth discussion of it here; however, here are some guidelines that work.

- Keep accurate records on a daily basis.
- Eat foods you enjoy but know when to stop.
- Enlist the support of friends and relatives.
- Weight yourself once a day in the morning before you consume food or liquids.
- Do not be so serious about things that you become depressed if you "blow it" occasionally.
- Do not expect to lose more than three pounds of per week. Chances are you will average one to two pounds per week. This is a tremendous amount of substance. Next time you are at a meat counter, ask the butcher for three pounds of fat. Have it put in a plastic bag, take it home, and look at it. You will have an idea about the amount of body fat you are losing. Seeing is believing.
- Expect about a seven to ten day lag time between when you start you weight management plan and when it actually begins to happen. Do not give up so soon.
- If possible, divide your total calories and meals into six or seven small meals. Eat something every two to three hours.
- Set realistic, long-term goals.
- Be patient. You can do it!

Because the body counts all food intakes as calories, it does not matter, technically, if the calories are in the form of steak or butterscotch candy. A calorie is a calorie.

What does matter is the nourishment provided by that food calorie. As an example: steak contains more nutrients than butterscotch candy, and steak is a better choice than candy.

For good health, which includes proper energy to perform daily tasks, tissue repair, growth, thinking ability and many other life factors, calories should provide at least the daily recommend allowance of all vitamins and minerals needed by the body.

Just as there are two basic components to weight loss: (1) lowering your food consumption and (2) increasing your activity level, there are two basic components to exercise as it relates to body weight and total fitness.

1. <u>Aerobic exercise</u>. This type of exercise requires you to move steadily for a prolonged period without rest. Many people think this means some kind of aerobic dance class is a mandatory ingredient. It is not.

Any continuous movement will suffice. That can be walking, jogging, running (on the road or on treadmills or elliptical machines), hiking, swimming, cycling (stationary and on the road), and rowing machines.

These activities uses large muscle groups, that burn more calories per minute than smaller muscle groups do, and done in a rhythmic, coordinated manner.

A major set back of this type of exercise is that it exercises primarily the lower body; therefore, one must enter into another type of exercise to tone and strengthen the upper body muscles.

We contend it is possible to follow a total body exercise program and derive all the benefits from one program. We will talk about this later in this manual.

Historically, fitness professionals recommend these activities relate to a large increase in the pulse rate.
The commonly recommended formula is to use the number 220 as the base number from which you subtract your age. That number is: Your maxim exercise target heart rate.

It is this heart rate you should not reach or exceed. It is dangerous to do so. Instead, take a percentage of the maximum heart rate that relates to your present level of condition.

The percentage, called an exercise heart rate, can range from a low of 50% (or less) of the maximum heart rate for anyone who never exercised and presently deconditioned, too as high as 80% to the maximum heart rate for anyone considered in "normal" health. The exercise heart rate relates to the intensity of your effort.

Once the exercise heart rate, therefore, the intensity is decided, one must decide how long to exercise with the pulse elevated at this level. Duration of exercise is relative to the present condition of the person doing the exercise.

Initially, you may be only able to walk for a period of 10 minutes before you become tired. Eventually, as you become in better condition you may be able to walk for periods up to one hour. Let a common sense prevail.

We recommend performing aerobic activities at "a talking pace". In other words, if you cannot hold a normal conversation at the same time you are walking, jogging, etc., then you are attempting a level of effort beyond your present, safe ability.

We also recommend that you pick the activity that places the less stress on the body. As an example, walking is less stressful than jogging or running. Less impact is placed on the body and the potential injuries associated with jogging or running does not materialize.

Studies show that with every running step one takes the impact upon stepping on the ground is equal to four times the body weight. It is no wonder that many runners are bandaged on various body parts because of running.

Check with your physician to determine your normal. The word normal is a confusing word because as it is generally used, normal compares to the average diagnosis of many people.

In our opinion, normal should relate only to your normal—given your past and present physical history and conditions.

Perform the exercises at a talking pace several times a week. The frequency can be from three to five days per week.

Related the frequency to the fatigue levels you feel at the end of each day.

The outlines we just covered are the four basic requirements one must meet as a state of aerobic conditioning. In short they are described as: (1) Movements that elevate the resting pulse, (2) that maintain it for a period of time, (3) using large muscle masses, (4) performed in rhythmic movement.

Keep these requirements in mind because, as you will later learn, any exercise program is aerobic in nature if it meets the above four requirements.

2. The second type of exercise and in our opinion the most valuable for losing body fat is <u>anaerobic</u> exercise. Anaerobic exercise consists of movements requiring muscle contraction against resistance.

The goal of anaerobic exercise is not to exercise for prolonged periods. It is to force muscles to work at a maximum level for a certain, predetermined amount of repetitions, and for a predetermined amount of sets.

This is the general approach, which we do not recommend. We will talk more about this later.

A set of an exercise is complete when one finishes the amount of repetitions required for that exercise. If you complete 10 repetitions and then stop, it is one set of 10 repetitions of that exercise. The set will take about 60 seconds to complete before the muscle fatigues.

Free weights (barbells and dumbbells) and high-tech equipment are the choices for this form of exercise. We feel anaerobic exercise is very productive and produces greater weight loss in less time than aerobic exercise.

Design a program to exercise <u>all</u> body segments rather than just the lower body as aerobic exercise typically accomplishes. More importantly, the total body exercise approach will create much more lean tissue (muscle tissue) on the body. Lean tissue requires more calories to maintain and nurture it than will adipose, fatty tissue.

The net effect is more calories burn within the same time, whether or not one is just sitting around, or when exercising. In addition, total muscle tone and improved physical shape appear and strength, flexibility muscular endurance, and cardio respiratory endurance improved together.

In other chapters, we will specifically outline the exercise approach to create a new, total body effect. We call this approach the *Time-efficient, Cost-effective* method.

Everyone Can Exercise Without Injury

A truthful and simple answer to the above question is: If there is movement, there is hope. This means that everyone can exercise without harm as long as there is the lightest amount of movement within the body.

There is no age restriction. There is no injury restriction. Everyone, from children to seniors, can make a commitment to exercise and to improve their life force. The important aspect is right attitude not age.

A commonly asked question by parents is "When should my children begin and exercise program?" Right attitude is a reflection to the child's initial expressions of interest to pursue exercise. It reflects the understanding that they must allow proper supervision and be willing to set a certain amount of time aside, on a weekly basis, to properly perform the exercise program.

A Dr. Lyle Micheli, a Director of Sports Medicine at Children's Hospital in Boston, says, *"The prevailing theory of weight training for children is not correct".*

Dr. Micheli put 18 boys and girls, ages 10 to 11 on a weight-training program for nine weeks. The strength of the upper and lower body each improved by more than 40 percent. This improvement contradicts the previous theory that: because youngsters lack abundant male hormones, before puberty, they will not greatly improve. We agree with him.

The use of exercise equipment by children, without proper supervision, is dangerous. There is a skill factor involved in using any exercise equipment, and it involves the ability to concentrate of the exercise movements.

Reports indicate that 35,512 weight lifting injuries resulted in visits to hospital emergency rooms.

Half of the injuries were in the 10 to 19 age groups. Most of these injuries occurred in the home.

A prime value of a child using high tech equipment is the safety factor. High tech machines are safer than free weights assuming the proper indoctrination.

Although exercise is perceived as difficult, it can be a pleasant experience for children. It will not be pleasant when perceived as punishment.

Children may lose interest quickly, and their exercise program should be rather brief. Six to Eight exercises are enough for ages up to 15. The exercises should cover major muscle structures. In general, you may follow the exact procedures recommended in this manual for children and adults.

Fitness gains, from the point of view of the child seem relatively slows in coming. All gains will be dependent on the genetic potential and age of the child. Before the onset of puberty, strength and size gains may be slower in coming when compared to the gains that will come during puberty. Patience is a prerequisite for any exercise program, for young and elders alike.

If the youngster begins to lose interest, vary the workout by adding new exercises and discontinue some of the original exercises. It is important that the body recuperate between workouts for maximum results to develop.

One final note about the youngsters exercises program and the effects it produces. Should a goal be to participate in a sport, especially a contact sport like football, exercise will strengthen the bones, tendons, ligaments, and muscles to a degree that may help prevent injuries.

Senior citizens experience improvements in strength, flexibility, muscle endurance, and cardio respiratory fitness that border on the astonishing. These improvements produce a better quality lifestyle resulting in fewer aches, pains, and improved energy.

Many senior citizens are involved in sports such as golf, bowling, and tennis. They spend much of their time working around the home, or performing volunteer work for various associations. These activities can create stress and sap energy levels. Exercise will help eliminate these problems.

Golf, tennis, and bowling are examples of "one-sided sports. Certain muscle groups accrue undue stress and impact while others are not stressed or exercised. This leads to pains and strains in areas such as the lower back, shoulders and legs.

It is common for seniors to have unbalanced strength levels, and this leads to other areas of the body compensating for the imbalance. Proper exercise can quickly bring the body back into balance and virtually eliminate the pains and strains.

Senior citizens mistakenly believe that they are beyond help, and believe they do not have time to exercise, or that it is dangerous to do so. Nothing could be farther from the truth.

No one is beyond help, no one! Seniors have nothing to lose, except low energy, aches, pains and poor performance in a favorite sport, and they have everything to gain.

Osteoporosis is a common problem occurring with advanced age. Experts agree bone thinning is preventable with regular exercise, a balanced diet that includes adequate calcium. Studies of astronauts under zero gravity conditions show that exercise in the absence of added stress to muscles and bones, does not prevent decalcification of bones.

When the senior exercise program is tailored to age, goals, needs, and lifestyle great benefits will be experienced; however, proper supervision, education, and motivation must precede all sane exercise programs.

Age is no barrier to good health. We owe it to ourselves, and our loved ones, to become healthy and fit.

Another segment of the population that sometime fears exercise is expectant mothers. Research indicates that expectant mothers can exercise safely, and in fact they ought to exercise to help insure a healthy pregnancy and a quick recovery after the child is born.

Physicians are now recommending exercise to help ease common problems, such as back strain, leg fatigue and low energy levels.

Of course, expectant mothers should get the approval of the physician before undertaking any exercise program either at home or in a fitness center.

The best option is to begin the exercise program before becoming pregnant, continue to exercise during pregnancy and begin again as soon as possible after delivery. Fitness is a way of life.

Pregnant women should not follow a so-called "high intensity" exercise program or exercise in hot environments.

Any woman with heart disease, hypertension, diabetes or depression <u>must be sure</u> to talk with her physician since the issues listed above, combined with exercise may be hazardous to both mother and fetus.

In summary:

- ✓ A safe and effective exercise program can be designed for everyone except those whose physicians do not recommend exercise because it is contraindicated for various reasons.
- ✓ As long as there is movement, there is hope!
- ✓ Youngsters can safely exercise and it will not cause any harm in any way—properly supervised.
- ✓ Discourage youngsters from over exercising.
- ✓ Exercise is beneficial for prevention and rehabilitation of injuries.
- ✓ Seniors can greatly benefit from properly supervised exercise programs.
- ✓ A natural extension of exercise for seniors is improved energy, strength, flexibility, muscle endurance, cardio respiratory fitness, and enhanced sports performance.
- ✓ Expectant mothers can safely exercise before, during, and after pregnancies. Proper supervision, education, and motivation are vital to insure the success and safety of an exercise program.

Before beginning an exercise program get the OK of your physician and discuss the design of your program with a fitness practitioner.

Fitness Training After 40 is it Worth the Effort?

Recently, three sisters—Joe-Anne, Carolyn and Melissa, each of them concerned about their parents health, asked me why so many people over 50 years of age feel that exercise is a waste of time. They wondered why parents feel at an advanced age, they are beyond help.

There is no one answers to this valid question. A general answer is that most of those in the 50 and beyond age group are victims of health and fitness misinformation.

A survey taken by the President's council on Physical Fitness and Sports, reported that "older" persons have formed many negative attitudes that are not correct. The report showed that:

- Older persons believe their need for exercise diminishes and eventually disappears, as they grow older.
- That they vastly exaggerate the risks involved in vigorous exercise after middle age.
- Older persons over rate the benefits of light, sporadic exercise; and,
- They under rate their own abilities and capacities.

Reports indicate that 60 percent of those over 45 reported that they attempted NO regular exercise. This may explain why so many senior citizens over 65 years of age see a physician more often that any other age group.

Recent evidence indicates that in addition to the general benefits of regular exercise, several major health problems are preventable or managed in part by an exercise program.

Coronary Heart Disease is a major cause of disability and death in the U. S. About one million people suffer heart attacks each year; 20 percent of these are immediately fatal. Exercising on a regular basis can greatly reduce your chance of succumbing to this deadly disease.

Hypertension or high blood pressure begins early in life and progresses with age. One of every six persons has hypertension, which is also a prime risk factor for coronary heart disease. Exercise is effective in reducing hypertension.

Arthritis is one of the major cripplers among Americans. There are over 100 kinds of arthritis and at least 31 million Americans suffer from one or more of them. Exercise is the cornerstone of arthritis therapy. It does not cure arthritis but it does allow for the control of symptoms.

Osteoporosis causes over 200,000 hip fractures annually, primarily to older women, and is a major cause of physical disability in old age.

Pain and shortened height, often accompanied by the so-called "dowager's hump" are major symptoms of advanced osteoporosis. Exercise can play an important role in relieving the anxiety and mild depression connected with osteoporosis.

Still not sold on the benefits of exercise? OK, here are important reasons to get off your duff. The following life changes usually related with aging improve with exercise.

Reduced muscle strength and endurance, loss of lean body mass and an increase in body fat, poor posture; reduced coordination and loss of agility, reduced joint mobility and diminished flexibility, loss of bone mass, reduced reaction time and decreased thinking ability. Is that enough reason to become active? We hope so.

Studies indicate that older people who exercise will experience quicker reaction time in processing information. The thinking ability of an older, fit person is greater that that of a 25 year old deconditioned person.

Every study indicates that life long exercise and exercise begun later in life can enhance all major components of fitness. There is hope for everyone; no one is beyond help.

Perhaps the greatest benefit of exercise is the sense of independence and self-esteem it provides. It will give you the courage to try many things that would be impossible without exercise.

The truth is we need not become victims of the perception of aging. All it takes is proactive commitment.

TESTING YOUR FITNESS IQ

When it comes to exercise, do you know the difference between fact and fiction? Discover your knowledge about exercise by taking the following true and false quiz, based on information adapted from the National Heart Lung and Blood Institute information (NHLBI).

QUESTIONS: TRUE OR FALSE?

1. Exercising gives you more energy.
2. All exercises do not give you the same benefits.
3. Exercising takes too much time.
4. The older you are, the less exercise you need.
5. You do not have to be athletic to exercise.

ANSWERS:

1. True. As their bodies get more in shape, most people feel exercising gives them even more energy than before they began exercising. Regular, brisk exercise can also help you resist fatigue and stress.

2. True. All physical activities can give you enjoyment. But only regular, brisk, and sustained exercises such as brisk walking, jogging, or swimming improve the efficiency of your heart and lungs, and burn off a lot of calories. Other activities do not give you these benefits, although they may give you other benefits such as increased flexibility or muscle strength.

3. False. Regular exercise does not have to take more than about 25 minutes to 40 minutes, three times a week. Once you have established a comfortable exercise routine, exercising becomes a natural part of your life.

4. False. With age, we tend to become less physically active, and therefore need to make sure we are getting enough exercise. In general, middle-aged and older people benefit from regular exercise just as young people do. Age need not be a limitation. What is important, no matter what your age, is tailoring the exercise program to your own fitness level.

5. True. Most brisk activities do not require any special athletic abilities. In fact, many people who found school sports difficult have discovered that these other activities are easy to do and enjoyable.

Can Exercise Improve Your Heart Health?

Several factors increase your risk for developing coronary artery disease and your chances of having a heart attack. Fortunately, exercise can help reduce or eliminate some of these risk factors, according to the NHLBI.

1. High Blood Pressure: Regular exercise is associated with lower blood pressure.

2. Cigarette Smoking: People who exercise vigorously and regularly are more likely to cut down or stop cigarette smoking.

3. Diabetes: People at normal weight are much less likely to develop diabetes. Exercise also decreases a diabetic's insulin requirements.

4. Overweight: Exercise can help individuals lose extra pounds or stay at ideal weight.

5. High Levels of HDL: High levels of HDL (one of the cholesterol carrying proteins in the blood called high-density lipoproteins) have are linked to a decreased risk of coronary artery disease. Studies have shown that regular exercise significantly increases the levels of HDL.

In summary, current evidence suggests that a moderate amount of regular, brisk exercise may reduce your chances of having a heart attack. Remember that even if you exercise, it is important to reduce or eliminate other risk factors so that you can lower your chances of having a heart attack as much as possible.

For your heart health: exercises regularly; stop or cut down on your smoking; control high blood pressure with proper treatment; cut down on fats, cholesterol, and salt in your diet; and reduce if overweight.

What If You Have Had A Heart Attack?

According to NHLBI, medical scientists do not know yet if regular, brisk exercise can reduce the risk of having another heart attack. However, regular exercise can improve the quality of one's life—how an individual feels and looks. It can help you do more than before without heart pain (angina) or shortness of breath.

If you've had a heart attack, you should consult your doctor to be sure you are following a safe and effective exercise program. Your doctor's guidance is particularly important because it could help prevent heart pain and/or further damage from overexertion.

What Are The Benefits And Risks Of Exercise?

Should you begin a regular exercise program? You can answer this question by considering the ways exercise can benefit you and weighing them against the possible risks.

Potential Benefits

1. More energy and capacity for work and leisure activities.

2. Greater resistance to stress, anxiety and fatigue and a better outlook on life.

3. Increased stamina and strength.

4. Improved efficiency of the heart and lungs.

5. Loss of extra pounds and help in staying at ideal weight.

6. Reduced risk of heart attack.

Potential Risks

1. Muscle and/or joint injuries.

2. Heat exhaustion/heat stroke on hot days (rare).

3. Aggravation of existing or hidden heart problems.

Before beginning an exercise program, check with your physician or qualified health practitioner.

WILL WOMEN DEVELOP MUSCLES LIKE MEN?

If women, when following a similar exercise program as that of a man, could develop muscles like a man, then the opposite would be true. Men, when following an exercise program similar to that of a woman, would develop a body like a woman.

Does any woman with a brain in her head believe that one?

Most women cannot! Some women can. Even if your genetic predisposition would allow you to build muscle, it is difficult to do so.

It is possible to get into fantastic shape without building large muscle size. Some women do have the potential for muscular growth. It can be traced to inheritance of above average levels of the hormone testosterone. This hormone stimulates muscular growth.

Other factors that contribute to potential muscular growth are: (1) origin and insertion of muscles (muscle length), (2) cross-sectional diameter (muscle width), (3) innervations (amount of nerve fibers attached to muscles), and (4) protein synthesis (increases hypertrophy of existing cells).

Another factor: mental disciplines, plays an important role in one's ability to exercise, be it for general fitness or athletic competition.

A woman must have adequate amounts of these factors (and others) to produce large muscle growth; most women don't, in fact, most men do not have the right combinations of these factors to assure above average muscle growth.

Some women are genetically gifted with esthetically pleasing bodily proportions and low body fat levels. Rare, these fortunate women may not need exercise to be in excellent condition.

The hormone estrogen is found in adequate amounts in females. It's slightly atrophying effect helps prevent masculine muscle growth.

It also has an effect on a woman sweating and accounts for the reason women sweat less than men during similar activities.

Therefore, it appears that exercise can produce many positive physiological changes in women, but large muscles are not a "normal" possibility.

If one is not interested in physique competition, yet gifted with the potential for large muscle size, even under the best of circumstances, does not happen over night.

If as one spends more time exercising, objectionable muscle growth seems to be taking place, adapt ones exercise program in a way as to preclude muscle growth.

Muscle tone, firmness and shape enhancement can be experienced without large muscle development.

Do not let misinformation or myths stop you from acquiring the health, fitness, and body you want and deserve. It will take some time however, do not expect over night miracles. Give yourself six weeks of dedicated hard work to begin to experience the wonders of a properly designed exercise program. You will be glad you do!

Should Women Approach Fitness Training Differently Than Men Do?

The manager of a woman's fitness center told us, "The only way to prevent women from getting muscles during exercise programs, is to have them breathe out deeply between repetitions."

For many years, women believed that they should perform different exercises than men. This misinformation was passed on by so-called health instructors there were certain exercises specifically for women and other exercises specifically for men. Women came to believe that, if they followed similar exercises as men, they would develop a masculine physique.

Contemporary women should know better than to believe misguided information like that, at least I hope they do. There is no need for men and women to do different exercises. They can if they wish, but there is no reason why they must.

Women's muscle structure closely resembles that of men. The functions of male and female muscles are the same. A woman's biceps performs the same movement as the biceps of a man; so do her leg muscles and other muscle groups in her body.

The function of a muscle group dictates the exercises to do to strengthen, firm and tone it. A manager of a woman's figure salon who told us startled us: "The only way to prevent women from getting muscles during exercise programs is to have them breathe out deeply, between repetitions."

The sad part of that statement is that she was sincere as she made the statement. There are probably hundreds of women who took instruction from this misguided soul, who passed the misinformation on to their children, family, and friends, continuing the circle of myth.

Rest assured the information in this book is safe to use (when following the directions) and unless you have inherited a body type that is already heavily muscled, there is no way that you will build massive muscles like a man.

As with exercise, women and men can follow the same diet. The diet recommendations in this book can help both women and men to lose unwanted body fat.

The scientific exercise principles offered in this book can benefit women and men and be adapted to the goals of both women and men.

It may come as a surprise to those reading this book that both men and women can follow similar exercise programs. Many authors do not point out this fact.

We feel it would be misleading and fraudulent to eternalize the myth of separate exercises for women and men.

LIES AND MORE LIES

One businessperson told us: "You'll never go broke under-estimating the intelligence of the public."

P.T. Barnum is credited with saying: "There's a sucker born every minute." It may have been he that said: "You'll never go broke underestimating the intelligence of the public."

In either case, the gullible public has shown those sayings right, by buying millions of dollars per year of useless products.

Witness an article reported by the Associated Press a few years ago: "Promoters of the Mark Eden Bust Developer and other devices that claimed to build bosoms and slim waistlines have agreed to pay a $1.1 million settlement in a mail fraud case."

The settlement involving Eileen and Jack Feather and four others was approved by U.S. District Judge Spencer Williams. The Feathers, who also owned the Cambridge Plan International, which promotes the Cambridge Diet, had sold the Mark Eden Bust Developer through mail order ads in magazines and newspapers.

The ads claimed the clam shaped discs could ad four inches to a woman's bust line in five days.

"A company spokesman said more than 4 million of the bust builders and midriff trimmer had been sold…indictments charging the couple and others involved in manufacturing and selling the exercise devices with mail fraud were issued in May 1982, but the Postal Service began its battle against the firms in 1965."

This story is a familiar one to fitness professionals who knock themselves out attempting to educate the public. Slowly, but surely, the educational battle is being won. People are learning to think and research products before parting with their earnings.

The list of useless, fraudulent products would fill a book the size of a dictionary. Suffice it to say that many, if not most, of the health related products on the market today is suspect.

If you have a tendency to shop for quick, easy answers to weight loss and fitness: Get ready to count yourself among the sucker born every minute group.

There are no magic lotions, potion, pills, and crèmes or bust developers and there is no tooth fairy. Surprised?

From our point of view, true health and fitness is mirrored by having the discipline, motivation, and patience to follow a balanced diet, and exercising to achieve above average levels of strength, flexibility, and endurance and below average levels of body fat.

PLEASANT PREGNANCY
EXERCISE AND PREGNANCY

Studies indicate that it can be safe to exercise before, during and after pregnancy.

Studies indicate that when following certain guidelines, it is safe to exercise before, during, and after pregnancy. Of course, you should first get your doctor's approval.

It is best to begin exercise before becoming pregnant; continue to exercise while pregnant and begin soon after the birth of your baby.

The American College of Obstetricians and Gynecologists have drawn up some guidelines prompted by the proliferation of home exercise programs by "non-professionals."

According to Dr. Art Ulene, who helped draw up the guidelines: "Pregnant women should not jog. Swimming, walking and stationary cycling are ideal."

Swimming may be the best choice of the three recommendations made by Dr. Ulene; because swimming involves more muscles than either walking or cycling, both of which are primarily lower body exercises.

In addition, an exercise program with free weights, high-tech machines or other equipment could be an improvement over swimming, walking or cycling, when the program is properly designed and supervised.

When you are trying to become pregnant or when you are pregnant, any exercise program should not be of the "high intensity" kind. Meaning: when the program is excessively difficult and requiring high levels of straining or very heavy breathing.

Here are some of the guidelines of The American College of Obstetricians and Gynecologists:

- Do not exercise strenuously for more than 15 minutes at a time.
- Maximum heart rate should not exceed 140 beats per minute.
- Do not exercise while laying flat on your back after the fourth month.

- Eat enough to compensate for the caloric output, above the additional daily calories advised during pregnancy.

Other recommendations during pregnancy and for at least one month after delivery:

- Exercise regularly—several times a week is better than intermittently.
- Don't exercise vigorously in hot, humid weather.
- Avoid jerky bouncy movements, such as aerobic dance.
- Avoid stretches or calisthenics that involve excessive flexing and extending: hormones released during pregnancy soften joint tissues, making them more susceptible to injury.
- Rise slowly to a standing position after doing floor exercises.
- Drink plenty of liquids before and after exercise. If you are over 30 and considering pregnancy, there are special considerations according to The University of Chicago Medical Center.
- Chromosomal abnormalities increase with age but can be diagnosed by prenatal tests such as amniocentesis or ultrasound.
- Older women should be screened for hypertension, diabetes, and plaque lining artery walls, all of which increase with age. These risks can be overcome if detected before pregnancy or in the early stages.
- The cardiovascular system and blood vessels are also examined before and throughout pregnancy.
- Before becoming pregnant, women should consult with her physician and work for six months to reach optimal condition; she should attain a proper diet, appropriate weight and good muscle tone.

In general, moderate exercise, under supervision, appears to be safe for all age groups; however, at least one study has indicated that "hard exercise" may make many young women temporarily infertile.

A study directed by Dr. Beverly A. Bullen of Boston University and published in The New England Journal of Medicine revealed that exercise could be a more common cause of infertility than experts had previously believed.

One researcher advised that women consider their exercise program if they are having trouble getting pregnant. Like many things in life, exercise can be a two edged sword.

The benefits are great, but it may not be advisable in all cases. Check with your physician. We would like to emphasize one aspect of exercise for pregnant, as well as non-pregnant women that are largely over looked.

That aspect is the speed-of-movement during an exercise movement. The faster the speed-of-movement, the greater chance of injury.

The speed-of-movement we are discussing is that taking place during exercise, with any exercise program. In simple terms, fast movement during exercise increases the impact forces on the body.

Think of it this way: if you had someone place his or her fist gently on your stomach and press on it hard, you would feel a certain amount of force or pressure "hitting" you.

Then, if you asked the person to reel back and punch you hard, you would feel a greater amount of force hitting you.

The differences in the impact forces you feel are caused by the speed-of-movement of the punch, when compared to just the pressure which lacks speed.

When performing an exercise program, always control the speed-of-movement. This approach eliminates the potential of damaging joints and muscles. When in doubt, slower movement rather that faster movement is desired.

BEFORE YOU BEGIN FITNESS TRAINING

Do not begin any exercise program before checking with your physician. Before you follow the strength training advice in this book, you should:

1. Advise your physician of your interest in strength training and get his or her O.K. to proceed.

2. Give serious consideration to NOT beginning any high-intensity, strenuous exercise program, if you are pregnant or have plans to become pregnant in the near future. Please review the chapter titled Pleasant Pregnancy, Exercise, and Pregnancy.

If you presently exercise and decide to begin strength training, use your present records to record your last complete workout. Include the total workout: sets, reps, weight used, sequence of exercises, and actual workout time.

This information will form the base of your test workouts in the future; we will use this workout to measure your improvements in six weeks.

Read the chapter titled: Balanced Strength Training. It is advisable to follow a program to eliminate any major muscular strength imbalances before you attempt flat-out, high-intensity training.

Get your muscle to body-fat ratio checked, accurately weigh yourself, and take all over body measurements. Use this information in the future, to evaluate your progress. Record this information on your improvement card in the back of this book.

PUMPING AEROBIC IRON

Exercise with resistance can enhance <u>total body fitness</u>. Aerobic dance as tradi-tionally practiced cannot.

Compared to the benefits of pumping iron, aerobic dance is a waste of valuable time. Especially if one has an injury.

Pumping iron, that is to say: exercise using high-tech equipment or free weights (under supervision), is the safest, most reliable and most versatile method of achieving aerobic fitness.

When properly designed, an aerobic weight program will also produce high levels of strength, flexibility, muscle tone and power.

Pumping iron is potentially more productive than aerobic dance, requires less skill training than swimming, produces less damage to the body than running and is less hazardous than bike riding on the open road.

Surveys indicate that 91 percent of women think aerobic dance is the best way to become fit. It is not. Often overlooked is that aerobic training does not produce total fitness. Its practice virtually ignores strength training.

We believe that LIFE IS NOT AN AEROBIC EVENT. For most people, strength specifically strength combined with muscular endurance is of more importance than heart condition.

The life-threatening heart attack is of such intensity, aerobic conditioning does not seem to help survival. We have often wondered what the survival ratio would be, if one conditioned the heart with short bursts of high-intensity exercise, rather than running.

Then, if the heart goes into trauma, could it ward off serious damage, because it is prepared for such a trauma? Perhaps we'll never know the answer.

In addition, there is a staggering difference in injury risk, between aerobic dance and weight training. Seventy percent of those instructing aerobic dance suffer injury.

Students of aerobic dance also sustain a high percentage of injuries. That is not said of weight training instructors or their students.

The basic principle of progressive fitness training is this: Supplies resistance to a contracting muscle and periodically increase the resistance as you become better conditioned.

Weight training allows precise increases in resistance. Aerobic dance does not; it periodically reduces intensity. This reduction comes about because of the weight loss typically experienced, by those watching their diets and while taking aerobic classes.

Here is why we feel aerobic classes can be deceiving: Aerobics programs become easier because most people use aerobics to lose weight. This means that each person starts the program with a total body mass and a specific weight of each arm, leg, upper torso, and hips.

Initially, performing movements that require one to lift arms and legs will have the same effect as weight training especially for those who are deconditioned. After all, lifting an arm or leg, upper torso or hips is lifting weight, the weight of the particular body segment.

As one "gets into condition" and loses body weight, it becomes easier to perform the movements. The aerobics program usually gets the credit for this perceived increase in fitness.

While some improvement take's place, the improvement is never attributed, to loss of body weight, which reduces the total body mass, as well as the weight of each body segment. One is then participating in the same aerobic class, using less resistance (loss of body fat).

Everything becomes lighter. It's as if you were weight training and began to use less resistance each workout. We have yet to meet a weight-training instructor who promises better results if you reduce the effort or intensity.

In effect, that is exactly what happens when one gets better, at aerobics.

There has been a feeble attempt to improve aerobic training by adding wrist and ankle weights or light dumbbells. The potential improvement is negated because most movements are done too fast (explosively).

So the weight is being thrown, not lifted, throughout the range of motion. Less weight lifted, less calories burned, less effort expended. All in the name of improved fitness, yet you cannot improve while decreasing the effort. Simple enough!

It is true that some research has shown it is not possible to reach an aerobic, steady state condition using free weights or exercise machines. Our opinion is that the research methodology was flawed, leading to erroneous conclusions.

The methodology was flawed. For example: the exercise sequence was wrong. Too many single-joint exercises mix with multi-joint movements in the same workout.

This is a mistake because it allows the aerobic heart rate to drop quite dramatically. Our research shows conclusively that: A properly designed strength-training program WILL IMPROVE AEROBIC CONDITIONING

As an example: Going from a leg press to a leg curl movement (in most cases) will allow the pulse rate to drop. We have found that some times, when the exercising person puts pressure on the rib cage (compression) this can alter the pulse and blood pressure dramatically.

Monitor this carefully. Be very careful of all exercises that put pressure on the rib cage area.

When designing an aerobic program using resistance, all exercises should be multi-joint movements for maximum aerobic benefit. Multi-joint movements use larger muscle masses, because they involve movement of more than one joint, and place a greater stress on the heart and oxygen uptake, resulting in the ability to maintain the targeted heart rate.

Single joint movements will not cause the required heart rate elevation, excepting for those very out of conditioned individuals or persons who have heart disease.

Contrary to popular belief, aerobic training with free weights or machines is possible and quite simple if you apply the rules for aerobic fitness.

The following are standard aerobic guidelines incorporated into a weight-training program.

(I) Choose movements that involve large muscle masses. Multi-joint exercises are best, for example: squats, leg presses, bench presses, chins, dips, pull downs, and rowing motions.

(2) Perform the movements smoothly and continuously and at a steady rhythm. We recommend a speed of movement of four seconds lifting and four seconds lowering. Do not pause at the start or finish of each movement.

(3) Determine the duration of the program according to the present fitness level. On average, 5 to 60 minutes of continuous activity is recommended, depending on ones starting fitness level.

Naturally, if one is much deconditioned, 5 minutes may be enough. It is recommended that one add to the above time a warm-up of five to 10 minutes and a cool down of five to 10 minutes. This warm-up is carefully observed, if one is working with a much-deconditioned person; it could be very taxing for this type of individual and may have to be counted a part of the aerobic timetable.

(4) Train two to five days per week. This is a general recommendation. Adjust it according to the intensity of the program and the level of condition of the client. Higher intensity means less total days committed to exercise, more devoted to recuperation.

(5) Gauge the intensity of efforts by pulse rate. This is often called a target exercise heart rate.

One way to arrive at your target heart rate, is to take the number 220 and subtract ones age from it.

Consider this a maximum heart rate. Then, depending on your present fitness level (check with your physician for advice), take 50 percent of your maximum heart rate (less for deconditioned persons) to 90 percent (for those in excellent condition. This will produce an exercise target heart rate.

If building total fitness is not your goal, it is possible to perform one exercise for the total time. After all, using a rowing machine or riding a bike is aerobic exercise, and in effect, each is one exercise, performed for one set for a specific period.

As previously indicated, there is more to total fitness than aerobic training can provide. Design a program that is enjoyable and varied and concentrates on multi-joint movements.

For body balance, you should not attempt to improve your superior areas. Exercise superior areas at a high level, but do not increase the resistance, reps, or sets. As lagging areas improve, work all areas with the same intensity.

Pumping aerobic iron is the safest, fastest, most precise and most time efficient way to build aerobic fitness. Best of all, strength, flexibility, muscular endurance, cardiorespiratory endurance, and power become enhanced.

EXERCISE SPECIFICS
THE PARTS OF THE WHOLE

The Beatles consisted of four parts: John, Paul, George, and Ringo. Each of them together comprised the complete Beatles.

Like the Beatles, each part of an exercise program must be in harmony with the others. It is mandatory when maximum results in minimum time are your goal.

Each specific unit making up the whole must be mathematically demonstrable. Only then is it possible to prove existing functional abilities, ones present health, and fitness level. It is not enough to justify improvements with the placebo effect of "feeling better." One must be able to quantify improvements.

The exercise tool one chooses to use for an exercise program is the foundation for fitness training.

We believe the proper use of high-tech equipment is potentially more beneficial, than other tools such as barbells (free weights). To give you the reasons for our preference, we must itemize a number of technical information, so bear with us.

The list of requirements we are about to enumerate is in the sense that, when one compares exercise tools, the tools meeting the majority of the requirements listed, would be the best choice for your exercise program.

HIGH-TECH VS FREE WEIGHTS AND IN-HOME EQUIPMENT

You may find this chapter laborious. We feel it is necessary to outline the differences between high-tech and non-high tech equipment.

Much of the equipment on the market is virtually useless. Only by knowing the basic principal of design and function—of not only the human body, but also equipment, can one decide the most time efficient means to exercise. With that goal in mind, we offer the following:

Once upon a time, the horse was the fastest form of transportation. If one's goal was to get from point A to point B, the horse was faster than walking.

Those without much time to waste took a horse, arriving quickly at the destination. Others has walked and eventually reached the destination.

Presently, the fastest form of transportation is a jet airplane.
If one's goal is to get from the East Coast to the West Coast, as quickly and safely as possible, the airplane is the best choice.

So it is in the choosing between non high-tech exercise equipment and high-tech equipment.

Non high-tech is today's equivalent of the horse. High-tech equipment is today's equivalent of jets. This is not to claim that, the proper use of free weights and other non high-tech equipment cannot be beneficial; however, for maximum results in minimum time there is no comparison.

The functions of the human body demands you use of an exercise tool design that includes certain biomechanical parameters lacking in non high-tech equipment. Function dictates design.

One major reason is the body stability provided by high tech equipment. We are all aware of the laws of force-counter force and the stresses placed on the body during exercise.

The support supplied to the body, when lying or sitting, during high tech exercise, helps stabilize the body, absorb counter force, and allows one to monitor and maintain proper body position.

This effectual eliminates unwanted stress to other body segments and eliminates injury during exercise.

Free weights, when used with various benches and seats can help modify some of the problems associated with force counter—force. However, not as well as machines do.

There are also many other bodily requirements for productive exercise, which only properly designed high-tech equipment can provide

Barbells were a quantum forward leap, because they allowed the basic requirement of productive exercise: Resistance, to be applied to a contracting muscle, with greater effectiveness than previously existing tools.

In truth, it does not matter to a muscle if one is lifting a 50 pound sack of sugar or a 50 pound barbell. The major difference is the comfort factor.

Performing a barbell exercise is easier. One major reason is one can grip it better than a sack of sugar. To the muscles doing the work, it is still 50 pounds. The amount of resistance used determines the amount of muscle fibers contracted.

Just as barbells were a quantum leap, so is high-tech equipment when compared to barbells. Application of resistance (the basic principle of progressive exercise and pro-active physical therapy) improves to a contracting muscle.

However, not all high-tech equipment incorporates all the requirements of maximum progress. Some of the requirements' one should consider are:

Positive and Negative Resistance

A properly designed exercise tool MUST provide two aspects of resistance. Resistance provided as one lifts and resistance must be supplied as one lowers the resistance.

Sometimes called concentric or positive resistance, this aspect takes place when one is contracting or shortening a muscle. Lowering resistance or eccentric, negative movement and takes place as one uncontracts or allows the muscle to lengthen.

Along with positive and negative resistance potentials, the ability to stretch and pre-stretch a muscle is essential with an exercise tool.

Pre-stretch and Stretching

Stretching is pushing or pulling a body part into a position temporarily exceeding the existing "normal" range of motion. It relates to the angels of the joints, muscles, and connective tissue.

Pre-stretching takes place when a muscle moves into a position of increased tension just prior to the start of a positive contraction. Pre-stretch has two effects that result in greater benefits:

(1) The muscle is elastic, just like a rubber band, and stretching it slightly, just before movement, actually produces elastic energy that can be used in the contraction and help you use more resistance.
(2) Pre-stretch ignites a nervous system stretch reflex that calls upon additional muscle fibers, for use in the upcoming movement

Now, we have established four requirements for full range, maximally productive exercise. They are:

1. Positive work: Lifting the resistance.

2. Negative work: Lowering resistance.

3. Stretching: A slight lengthening of a muscle groups.

4. Pre-stretching: Takes place in a slightly extreme range just before the stretch. It must be done carefully and with minimal speed.

5. Balanced Resistance and Variable Resistance

As muscles contract and move through a range of motion, they do so with varying degrees of movement and strength potentials.

This is a natural consequence of muscular contraction and human movement.

You are aware it is possible to handle more resistance in some exercises than others. You may not be aware that as one performs an exercise, the muscles involved, are also changing strength levels as they move.

That's one reason why some positions of a movement feel easier than others, although the weight remains constant.

Because muscles have a variable strength potential as they move, it logically follows that, the resistance should vary according to the actual muscle strength potential.

This is termed automatically variable resistance when incorporated into a high-tech machine design. When referring to the various muscle groups and varying strength potentials, it is termed balanced resistance.

High-Tech equipment should provide automatically variable resistance and balanced resistance. The resistance should vary automatically, and according to the strength potential, as one move through a range of motion. With barbells, the resistance does not vary.

We have now established, two more requirements for a superior exercise tool, neither of which barbells supply:

6. Balanced resistance: Resistance that is neither too light nor too heavy.

7. Automatically variable resistance: The resistance varies within the range-of-motion and in accord with a particular muscle group's strength potential.

8. Unrestricted Speed-of-Movement

Although it should be possible to perform exercise movements at various speeds for high intensity contractions, throwing the resistance is not beneficial. However, unrestricted speed of movement is a requirement. Barbells supply this requirement as does high-tech equipment.

For best results, perform movements rather slowly. As an example: the positive portion of the movement should take about 4 seconds, the negative portion about 4 seconds (as a safe example).

By controlling the movement, the muscle is contracting always. A fast speed of movement to is potentially dangerous.

It compounds the force. First, at the sudden, jerky start. Then again, as the resistance bangs into a body part, at its final destination point.
If a muscle is not prepared for the beginning sudden jerk, injury is a possibility.

9. Resistance In The Fully Contracted Position

Unless resistance exists in the position of full muscular contraction, it is impossible to exercise a muscle through its full range-of-motion. That is basic premise of full-range exercise.

Many but not all high tech machines provide proper variable and balanced resistance, in the position of full muscular contraction. Other forms of exercise tools, such as barbells, do not. Therefore, it would indicate that resistance is not supplied full-range, only partial-range. This lessens the exercise potential.

For instance, in the two-arm curling motion using a barbell, there is no affective resistance supplied to your biceps muscle in the fully contracted position.

With properly designed high tech equipment, there is resistance in this position.

We already understand that resistance, properly supplied, is the key to maximum results in exercise.

10. Direct Resistance

When possible, resistance must exist directly to the muscle under contraction to insure best results. Two similar exercises we can compare are the two-arm chinning movement and a high-tech pullover machine.

When performing a two-arm chinning movement, you will provide resistance to the latissimus dorsi and biceps of the upper body (among other muscles). During the movement, the biceps will
fatigue before the larger, stronger back muscles.

Therefore, you would not exercise the latissimus dorsi muscles as effectively, because of the weak link.

High tech pullover machines supply resistance of a higher quality to the latissimus dorsi muscle groups. By removing the weak link, in the two arms chinning movement and applying the resistance pads to the upper arms near the elbows' one works the back muscles thoroughly.

When one fails to continue movement, due to muscular fatigue, the primary muscles fail, not a weaker link in the chain.

11. Full-Range Resistance

Muscle contraction provides movement of one or more body segments. These segments have what can be termed a complete or full-range possibility.

Ideally, one should be able to exercise a body segment through a full-range of movement. Naturally, an injury may prevent this from happening; however, the goal is too to improved full-range movement.

This requirement rotary form movement is the hardest to visualize. In simple terms, it is: Resistance moving on a common axis with a body segment being moved by muscle contraction.

One excellent invention in the history of exercise is a device called the cam. It is a cam that allows the experienced of maximally productive exercise.

In simple terms, the function of a cam is as follows:

A cam redirects resistance, so it travels in the same strength curve as the exercised body segment. The resistance is re-directed to travel in a rotary motion and in the same strength curve of the moving body segment. At the same time the resistance is directly OPPOSITE the intended movement.

This assures resistance, typically provided by a weight stack. The lifting of the weight stack takes place through either cables or chains attached to it.

The cables or chains attach to the cam system and as the cam rotates, the cables or chains wrap around the cam. The radius of the cam that the chain wraps into varies.

The distance from the center mark of the cam radius, to the point where the chain touches as it wraps, determines the varying (and supposed balanced resistance). The touching point of the chain is directly opposite the direction of muscle contraction.

Barbells and some other forms of exercise equipment do not supply resistance in this manner. They supply resistance in a straight line manner, always directly down toward the ground, always depending on gravity.

Effective resistance is when you are moving the barbell vertically, directly opposite the pull of gravity.

A cam changes straight-line resistance (gravity) into rotational resistance. This allows the resistance to travel in a curve always pulling directly away from your movement.

Because barbells and some exercise machines can meet only some of the requirements we have listed, it follows that high-tech has the potential to improve one's fitness results.

The QUALITY of the resistance is the final determining factor, determining which exercise tool provides best results.

Calisthenics and aerobic dance supply minimal resistance (arm legs, torso, and lower body).

Gymnastics type exercise can be more productive because a larger body mass is moved; therefore more resistance is handled by muscle groups.

Barbells, pulleys and the like are more productive than either of the two mentioned because, resistance adjusts according to one's fitness level.

REPETITIONS

Repetitions are a personal decision.

The first several repetitions are looked at as a warm up.

The middle amount are preparing the muscle to fatigue.

The final repetitions are preparation for complete muscle fatigue.

How many reps adequately prepare ones' muscles for safe, affective contractions and potential results? The answer is: it depends.

It depends on ones previous physical history, present injuries, age, circulatory system, neurological system, present fitness level and other factors.

The variance of these factors between humans, make it all but impossible to suggest a specific individualistic repetition protocol.

The idea of sets was advanced in a "scientific" way years ago, by a study recommending 3 sets of 10 reps.

In the exercise definition, a set would represent one exercise performed for a certain number of repetitions before stopping the exercise. If one were to perform the exercise again, it is the second set, etc.

Those initial recommendations have altered over the years, primarily by magazines specializing in body building advice. Every conceivable amount of total sets, reps and workout days are recommended since then.

Most of the recommendations preached a more is better approach. Not scientific reasoning. Just the idea that if three sets work well, then 12 sets will work better. Other studies have not defined an exact protocol of reps or sets.

Presently, people pick a number of sets and if results are not forth—coming, the more is better concept is applied. The total sets are increased.

Eventually, after wasting much valuable time, those following this approach quit exercise entirely or remain satisfied with minimal progress.

There is no "absolute" amount of repetitions that are right for everyone. Your personality and psyche, will guide you to the amount that feels safe and enjoyable to you.

What I find produces maximal fitness in minimum time is using a number of 10 repetitions as the least amount to perform, and when you can perform 15 repetitions, that is the cut off point.

Repetitions and Genetic Numeric Rhythm

For reasons we cannot explain, many perhaps most people, want to select a repetition count they like the "feel of," meaning: a certain number of reps feel good (therefore pleasant) to some and another number feels good to others and they prefer that amount.

We have therefore concluded: the human body has a built in rhythmic numeric system that, in the exercise sense, feels pleasant and guides one to want to achieve a certain number of reps. Then the system begins to signal for muscle contraction and mental shut down.

Some people prefer low repetitions: six to ten; while others prefer to work with less weight and in higher reps: 10 to 20 repetitions. You may have a slightly different numeric system. Keeping in mind the individual numeric system, let us establish a base line for proper safe exercise.

(1) To prevent injury, we must select a minimum amount, which will allow a proper warming up of the musculo-sketal system.

We know if we use very low reps, such as two or three reps for the rep blue print, it could cause injury. If one attempts to lift too much weight too soon the body structure is not prepared.

(2) The minimal number 8 works well for most people. Therefore, we must select a resistance that will allow, at least, a safe MINIMUM of eight repetitions. Then we are sure the structure is safely prepared for the exercise. In addition, one's mind has had time to focus on the task and the resistance is not too heavy.

(3) Having established a safe minimum, we must establish a rationale maximum amount of reps; this maximum is the signal to increase the resistance.

In practice, this means a number of reps above the minimum, which will allow one to achieve a maximum without becoming mentally tired. As you probably know, the mind may quit short of muscle failure. However, failure is failure.

Our recommendation is to select a guide number as a starting point and stopping point. Later, you can select a rep count that is more comfortable.

The important element is to select a safe minimum and a reasonable maximum.

Sets

The questions of how many sets you should perform is a controversial one. We conducted extensive research into this question and, to be brief, we recommend the following for standard exercise procedure:

If you are much deconditioned, use a warm-up set. Use about 50% of the resistance you will use during the exercise program.

Allow a rest until the pulse normalizes. Then, follow the warm-up set with a one set to complete muscular failure, emphasizing excellent style of performance.

If one is normally healthy, use one set to failure, following the repetition guides we have presented.

When the speed-of-movement is controlled, there is no chance of injury.

SPEED-OF-MOVEMENT

Speed-of-Movement is the most dangerous aspect of exercise. Over training only causes fatigue and possible lack of improvement
It may cause great trauma and even death.

In an exercise sense, think of it this way. If a medium framed person is lying on his or her back, a weight it is possible to place something on the chest area without any damage. Let us say a 50-pound barbell.

Muscle and bone structure support the barbell. There is no speed-of-movement in the equation. No impact force! Now, pick up the barbell and drop it from arm's length on to the person's rib cage area. What would happen? Correct, severe damage to the body.

What changed in the equation? The person was the same one whose chest could support the barbell. The barbell is still 50 pounds.

Only one factor changed the introduction of speed-of-movement or acceleration. The barbell accelerated to a speed of X miles per hour. The impact force was the resulting cause of the damage.

One can see that weight or mass by itself may not cause injury. Muscles, bones, tendons and ligaments may manage the resistance...Unless excessive speed-of-movement is introduced into the parameters.

In an exercise sense, speed-of-movement MUST be controlled.

Rapid movement during exercise produces momentum, not results. Explosive movements produce momentum, not results. Momentum produces potential impact forces.

Throwing weight through the air is not a test of strength. It is a test of acceleration. A test of acceleration in a racecar is fine, in exercise, not!

Exactly what is a safe speed-of-movement? In standard exercise (not advanced procedures), lifting to a count of four seconds and lowering to a count of four is safe and affective.

Advanced training, require lifting to a count of four and lowering to a count of two.

In our super-advanced Primordial Principle, seven seconds in each direction is recommended (this concept is discussed on the 120 minute audio cassette and CD titled: Secrets of Advanced Exercise)

When in doubt, slow the movement down, rather than moving faster.

REST TO WORK RATIO

Humans must eventually rest. Sleep is a survival requirement. Fatigue sets in quickly for one whom suffers with injuries. After the biochemical damage created by exercise, the body must recuperate.

This recuperation takes place within the actual workout itself and between exercise bouts.

Depending on ones present health and fitness level and actual injuries, the rest period is essential and varies individually.

As important as the work to rest ratio within the exercise program is, the rest period between visits is most important.

Presently, most fitness enthusiasts use the three visits per week protocol. Our studies indicate this approach to be inferior to two visits per week. Ideally, four or five days rest between visits works wonders when compared to the three visits' scenarios.

The higher the intensity of effort, the more one infiltrates the body's recuperative system. It then follows that more rest required. It is that simple.

If you are not improving on a steady basis, something is wrong with your approach to exercise or daily lifestyle. Most of the time, the culprit will be over training, and that you are not completely recuperating between exercise visits.

Strength versus Flexibility

There can be no progress, without a break in traditions. Otherwise, we would still be living in caves. So, it is in the exercise field. Without challenging tradition, there can be no break-through.

Many professionals and fitness enthusiasts, especially those in the therapy arena, strongly argue that flexibility is more important than strength. That point of view is popular among coaches and athletes alike.

For decades, women have overlooked the value of strength training. Men over shadow women in the strength arenas.

In practical everyday living, women become the target of thugs, whose only line of offense (other than weapons) is usually superior strength or size, which usually accompanies strength and visa versa.

Women take self-defense classes to improve the odds. In our opinion, the odds would be more in a woman's favor, if she improved her strength.

The self-confidence, accompanying increased strength is sufficient to project the required confidence, alertness and courageousness needed to walk the streets.

We believe strength is of more value than flexibility. We offer the following intellectual ammunition deserves attention.

Imagine the physical stature of Woody Allen. Put him alongside Arnold Schwarzenegger. Then, picture Woody attempting to twist Arnold's arm at the shoulder, to see how flexible Arnold is.

Ask Arnold to do the same to Woody's arm. Whose arm do you think would break and why?

After you accompany Woody down to get his arm in a cast, will you advise him to take more yoga classes or perhaps to tag along with Arnold to the weight room.

The importance of strength versus flexibility to prevent and rehabilitate injury has ramifications far beyond hypothetical arm-twisting.

Rather, it goes to the heart of health and fitness training, athletic training, rehabilitation, physical therapy and injury prevention.

The American economy loses approximately $40 billion every year, because of musculo-sketal problems, related to back problems alone. Injuries that affect 80% of the work force at some time in their lives.

We use the Woody and Arnold image, to illustrate the body's ability to handle complex biomechanical demands without injury, is better served by building adequate and well-balanced strength, rather than by simply becoming more limber.

Properly conditioned muscles can with stand the long-term stress placed upon them, by everyday tasks and the tremendous amount of sudden impact force. Which is simply:

The weight of an object (your arm, leg, head, or torso), multiplied by the speed of its movement, when pushed, pulled, twisted or slammed into an object.

When the force of your golf swing, tennis serve or running gait are no longer absorbed by your muscles, which act as shock absorbers, the impact transfers to bones and joints. Injury is the very predictable result.

The flexibility of a yogi will not be able to prevent impact forces from applying torque to a body segment.

Back problems are a particular problem for every class of American worker. To understand its source, we need only visualize the stress we place on the back, almost every minute we are not laying down, in a stress free position.

Sitting all day in your office chair or standing at your counter, can be likened to walking around, carrying a five pound object (a dumbbell as an example), which you keep in a perpetual position biceps curl, hand help halfway to shoulder. Despite the objects relatively lightness, after a while the strain will begin to show.

At the end of such a day, you will be reaching for the aspirin (or scotch) bottle seeking relief.

The back takes on this stress. It must constantly fight against gravity to hold your torso erect. The effect of a WEAK back, most commonly seen in the elderly, whose back muscles can no longer support the torso weight erect, as gravity pulls the torso forward into a stooped position.

This problem is offset by a back-strengthening program.

With backs and other body segments not meant to handle the upright strain humans put on them daily, any exercise therapy or rehabilitation protocol, without strength as its central focus, is doomed to utter failure.

While passive therapies such as, stretching, massage and the like to nothing to improve strength, each has a limited role to play.

They do nothing to alter the structural capacity of the muscles to absorb impact stress or prevent unwanted torque around body joints.

Proper strength training will provide adequate structural integrity.

Equally important as muscle strength is muscular balance. This is thought of as the relative function and balance of one side of the body compared to the other. This applies in a side to side as well as a back to front plane.

Do not think being an active sports participant will improve the situation. The opposite is true. Witness the over developed and dominant body segments of golfers, tennis players and bowlers (as examples), it is no accident the display poor posture and has back, shoulder, elbow, and wrist problems.

Unfortunately, most of them accept joint pain and poor posture as the cost of sports participation. Lack of strength, not lack of flexibility is their problem.

The problems, when compounded by well meaning therapists and trainers, who put these athletes on an exercise program without thinking through the problems.

If we agree that muscular imbalance exists and is caused by one side of the body being more dominant than the other, then it would make sense to design a workout program to focus on NON-DOMINANT areas and ignore the already dominant side. At least until the weaker areas improve and are in closer relationship to the superior areas.

But, nnoooo, instead, programs are designed which exercise both sides, thereby improving each side, but doing nothing to improve functional muscular balance. Each area improves and the imbalance ratio stays the same.

Rather than eliminating the problem, most fitness and therapy programs continue on the right track but heading in the wrong direction.

High-Tech exercise machines and new concepts of exercise allow one to achieve maximum fitness in minimum time; however, proper use of this equipment and application of new techniques to improve fitness and functional ability become ignored by many. Instead, they continue the dogma of the past, never thinking about a new approach.

Myths, misconceptions, old wives' tales, and outright lies continue and everyone loses.

If more times are given to proper strength training, work injuries, daily activity injuries and sports related injuries would be dramatically reduced or totally eliminated.

THE MATHEMATICAL BASIS
OF GUARANTEED PROGRESS

"For whatever deserves to exist deserves also to be known, for knowledge is the image of existence; and things mean and splendid exist alike."

Francis Bacon
(1561 1626) English essayist, philosopher.

In the early 1970's, to measure exercise progress, we began to use simple, previously established mathematical formulas. We decided to use the standard formula for Work, which is Work Equals Force Times Distance.

We renamed it: Units of Progress. Later we renamed it Units of Muscular Contraction.

Now we called it The Life Force Index.

The Life Force Index is to us, the most significant insight to assuring progress. Everyone interested in time efficient exercise finds it especially beneficial.

Including new concepts into an exercise program is always a battle between prior knowledge, some of which trickle down generation to generation, coupled with a fear that the new ideas will not work.

This pulls in two directions at the same time. Our recommendation is to try new ideas. After all, if they do not work you will know it soon enough and you can always return to previous models.

The Life Force Index is a mathematical application of long established exercise ideas that include three components: (1) A set (or more) of an exercise; (2) The amount of resistance being used; (3) The repetitions performed.

We are not considering the speed-of-movement. We are assuming you are intelligent enough to monitor speed-of-movement.

In formula, it is I=R. X. R (Improvement Equals Resistance Multiplied by Repetitions).

Let us dissect a typical exercise as presently performed by most people. Then, we will examine what the average trainee, thinks is progress. Most people believe the workout in which they increase resistance marks progress.

We will use only one exercise as the example but the concept applies to any number of exercises and the total workout.

Assume we are analyzing an exercise done during a Monday workout:

The exercise is leg extensions, 90 pounds of resistance is used and 10 repetitions are performed before muscular fatigue is reached. Not one more repetition is possible.

We get a factor of 900 units of work by multiplying 90 times 10.

Now, let us move into a workout performed on another day and let's make believe you've decided to increase the resistance.

We have already stated that, during the previous workout, 10 repetitions were attained using 90 pounds of resistance. Now, we're going to increase the resistance by 10 pounds, a typical increase by most people.

If one could do 10 repetitions with 90, it will not be possible to perform 10 repetitions with 100 pounds. Let's say eight repetitions are reached and not one more could be performed.

Eight reps multiplied by 100 equals a factor of 800. Is the number 800 larger or smaller than 900?

Obviously, if one performs 900 units of work on one day, and performs 800 units of work on another day, less work is performed and the workout is virtually wasted.

Possibly, the person might have performed eight reps with 100 during the previous workout, if they had decided to try it.

Usually, the cycle continues on this order: Increasing resistance equals decreasing repetitions. How can anyone claim any strength or muscular endurance, muscle tone or muscle's size improvements have taken place?

It is much like standing in the middle of a room, having a goal of reaching the far wall, then continuing to run in place. Something IS taking place; something is going on, but nothing productive is taking place.

For exercise improvements to take place, we must constantly strive to improve the units of work. It is really quite simple. Take these measurements every workout.

There is only one rational way of accomplishing this goal. Suppose, when exercise resistance is increased, it increases in minimal amounts, allowing one to at least match, preferably EXCEED, the previous work factor.

If in the example we are using, you increase the resistance by say, 2 1\2 pounds (or less) instead of 10 lbs. Here is what would happen.

Because the increased resistance was minimal, it will feel to ones mind, as it is almost non-existent. To the muscles, the increased load will feel like a feather.

We have successfully bridged the gap between mind and body. One will not feel like "it's too much," either in the psychological sense, or the physiological sense.

In almost cases, in almost each exercise, improvements take place and mathematically proven correct. Most importantly, improvements take place workout to workout.

The major problem, of increasing the resistance without any rational guideline is that it will take several workouts or several weeks, to match or exceed a previous workload.

To prove this to yourself, just take a mathematical look at a friend's workout card. You will find much numbers when calculated, as indicated, will amount to wasted workouts. Something took place. Yet nothing of benefit took place.

Get the picture?

The secret to more strength, muscular endurance and cardiorespiratory fitness, lies in applying mathematics to ones' workouts.

The secret to sustained improvements in exercise or physical therapy is the application of mathematics exercise.

You must increase resistance in very small amounts.

Depending on the mass of muscle involved, meaning: origin, insertion and cross-sectional diameter, etc., some muscles can handle slightly larger increases than others can. One must experiment a little to find out.

How much of an increase? That depends on factors such as just mentioned, plus, neuromuscular innervations, present strength level (the stronger one is, the harder it is to get stronger), mental strength (ability to keep on keeping on) and one's willingness to follow advice.

If one increases resistance in small amounts, progress will continue steadily upward slope. When one uses too much resistance, progress WILL plateau for long periods of time.

We have all settled for minimal results, by thinking progress is measured in minuscule amounts. We think in minuscule amounts because we have used illogical methods of exercise.

Change this approach by evaluating progress in mathematical ways. Once one begins to measure in meaningful ways, fitness results happen in meaningful ways.

Results! That is what The Life Force Index represents.

THE TIME FACTOR AND
ITS RELATIONSHIP TO EXERCISE

"If time was not a moving thing…"

The time factor is an important element in exercise. Time efficiency is of vital importance, for time management and producing maximum results in minimum time.

Time efficiency and time management are interchangeable. A properly designed program is time efficient when time management is in place.

When we ask ourselves, what is the MINIMUM amount of exercise required to reach the stated goals, we automatically enter into time efficiency and time management.

However, once a total program is decided, time becomes even more important. Enhanced results happen by increasing the relative intensity of the program.

Meaning: constantly striving to perform work in a shorter time, without sacrificing proper exercise style or increasing the speed of movement within each repetition.

Here is an outline of a program in a time\work relationship sense:

Suppose, a program of 8 total exercises are selected and a repetition system is outlined, as is a speed-of-movement frame work.

For instance, during the first complete workout, we record a supposed time of 30 minutes.

That time factor is one basis for future evaluations of improvement. Reps, weight, and speed-of-movement are also indicators. We are focusing specifically on the relationship of exercise to rest time.

If a speed-of-movement of six seconds is used for each rep, which is: 2 seconds to lift and 4 seconds to lower, a total time for each rep is 6 seconds. We are using the 2\4 count as an example, because many people use this count.

If each rep takes six seconds and one completes an average of 10, reps per exercise: that is a total of 60 seconds per exercise.
Multiplying 60 seconds per exercise by 8 total exercises, we get a time factor of 480 seconds or 8 minutes for the completed program.

Where was the balance of the 30 minutes spent? Unless one is extremely deconditioned and required much rest, the time is wasted. The explanation we just outlined was a rather long-winded way, of focusing on the importance of keeping an eye on actual exercise time.

One can see for instance that within the example 30-minute workout much time may be wasted.

Improvements in functional ability and physical fitness are greatly enhanced by attempting to lower the rest time between exercises (up to a point).

If you change nothing but this factor, improvements escalate. One need not necessarily lift more weight or perform more reps to show a marked improvement in exercise, as is commonly thought.

Another way to manipulate time is a concept we call Time Warp Training. For instance: if you are do not like lifting what feels to you as too heavy a weight, you can get better results by shifting the time and automatically requiring less weight.

Suppose you are presently lifting a weight to a count of 2 and lowering it to a count of 4 (this is the most common approach we've observed but don't recommend).

This represents a total repetition time of 6 seconds. Try changing the Time Warp factor by lifting to a count of 4 and lowering to a count of 2.

That speed, although it is still 6 second's total, will produce a more intense contraction.

The reasons are, by slowing the lifting movement; one is forced to contract the muscle more intensely and by lowering quickly (but safely) the rest time between contractions shortens by half. Initially, you will not achieve the 10 reps you did, with your usual resistance. This will prove the point we are making.

Later in this book, we will outline why we recommend lifting a weight slower than one lowers it. Time affects the total workout. Each element, such as: (I) Actual exercise time. (2) Total elapsed time. (3) Each single rep and total reps. (4) Rest periods. (5) Recuperation.

To manage a Strength Program, you must manage time and you must manage the following:

1. The total exercises.

2. Follow a safe and productive speed-of-movement in each direction, both lifting and lowering, (call it positive and negative movement or eccentric and concentric, if you prefer).

3. Format a minimum amount of repetitions and a maximum off repetitions, for each body segment.

4. Select an initial sequence of exercises. Then, do not repeat that sequence again in a workout. Instead, mix the exercises every workout. Several weeks later, for test and evaluating a workout, follow the exact initial sequence and use the initial starting resistance for the test workout; however, this time continues to work to absolute muscular failure within each exercise.

5. Select the proper rest between each set of exercise. Initially, is calculated on the starting fitness level. Then, each visit; reduce the rest time between exercises and always within your ability to continue.

6. Use the Units of Progress Index to monitor progress.

7. Decide the amounts of days rest between visits. We recommend resting four days between exercise visits if possible. Otherwise, use a Monday Thursday or Tuesday and Friday workout schedule. If Saturdays will work for you, use a Wednesday and Saturday schedule.

ACCENTUATE THE NEGATIVE
FITNESS WITHOUT "LIFTING" WEIGHTS

Many people think that injuries prevent one from "lifting" weights or using any high-tech equipment in the exercise program. This is not true.

Since we base our approach to exercise on rational and proven ideas, we prefer to eliminate traditional approaches and produce results as quickly as possible. For those who exercise on a consistent basis, injuries may be part to the game.

One of the simplest and quickest ways of improving functional ability of an injured body segment is a system of exercise called: Negative Training.

In the January 1973 issue of Iron Man magazine, an article titled, "Accentuate the Negative," written by Arthur Jones, outlined a method of strength training virtually unheard of then.

For the purposes of this chapter, lifting resistance is thought of as a "positive" movement and lowering it is called "negative" movement. The idea touted the effects of focusing on the negative or lowering of resistance, rather than the positive or "lifting" of it.

Back then, exercise was a method of lifting resistance, with every effort judged by how much one could lift. Little or no thought is given to the possibility of improvements, based on the lowering of resistance.

This lifting approach is still the commonly accepted way to perform physical therapy exercise. The focus on a patient's ability to lift (or not lift) a weight, is one of the reason some therapists prefer to provide passive therapies for weeks, rather than an immediate exercise program.

After reading Mr. Jones' article, we immediately began studies to test the concept. As usual, we tried the concept on several adventurous training partners and ourselves. Strength improvements began immediately. We were noticeably stronger starting with the second workout.

There was one major problem with this exercise method. One becomes so strong at lowering resistance; it soon takes several people to help lift the resistance, into the position of muscular contraction.

Then one "uncontracts" the involved muscles and lowers the resistance. Another problem is, it takes its toll on your training partners, and they are doing a workout with you. We are talking in the context of a healthy person performing this concept, not an injured person.

This problem, will not arise when one is training a physical therapy patient, given the goal of returning the person to only "normal" functional ability.

Following is a summary of our method of adapting this approach.

Negative exercise concentrates on the movement that starts an exercise in the position of full muscle contraction. Another person must lift the resistance into position. Then focused control is used to lower the resistance.

Let us use the curling motion as our example. The movements, starting from the shoulders, or contracted position, to a position, where the arms are fully straight. Some have referred to this movement as the uncontraction of muscles.

We are talking about helping an injured person, to perform this exercise safely. Use caution at all times. Two major concerns are: (1) What is the active range of motion and, (2) How much resistance is used?

Test the active range of motion by having the patient attempt to move from a position of full extension, to one of full contraction.

It is assumed, as an example, if the person can bend an arm from a straight position, to a half way to shoulder position, then the active range of motion is, say: 90 degrees.

Yet, if the patient is helped to raise the arm to shoulder level, they may be able to move it, under control, from the shoulder to a straight-arm position. Therefore, it is obvious the range has a greater potential, IF there was enough strength to curl the weight of the forearm and hand, upwards towards the shoulder

So, depending on how one evaluates range of motion, one could test either way, attempting to lift or lower a body segment.

It is also obvious that, although the muscles are unable to lift the weight of the forearm and hand, the muscles are capable of lowering the weight. This phenomenon is noticeable in all body segments. One can lower more resistance than one can lift.

Some studies reported the strength differentiation between muscles lifting and lowering weight is 40 percent. In our experience, this percentage difference is incorrect.

We found the difference to be much greater, depending on which body segment, muscle groups and range of motion were tested. For discussion sake, let's agree with the figure of 40 percent.

Negative training takes advantage of this inherent strength difference. As for the question of: How much resistance is used? We recommend an educated guess, erring on the low side when in doubt, rather than using too much resistance. It's always possible to use more resistance during another visit.

Initially, an injured person may find the weight of the forearm and hand (in this example), as heavy enough to attempt to lower. There is no absolute recommendation we can make, other than to take you time testing for negative strength potential.

To continue: Let us say you have decided the person can use a 20 lb. weight for the exercise. Now, you must educate the person as to your expectations of proper exercise procedure.

Here is proper exercise procedure: Using a guideline of 1 set of 10 repetitions.

He or she will carefully move the resistance, with your help, into the fully contracted position. Then, to a count of 10, one is to control the movement from the shoulder to a straight-arm position. The control must be slow and special effort made not to move into a hyper-extended position, as the arm is straightened.

If you guessed right about resistance, the first several repetitions will seem incredibly easy, (assuming there is no high pain level).

Then, as the muscle groups tire, the resistance will reduce the strength of the muscles with each succeeding repetition

About halfway into the 10 reps, you'll notice the movement may begin to speed up, especially in the midrange position. It is at this point that, you should watch for any unwanted speed of movement

You must remind the patient to focus and remain in control. For safety sake, stand close to the person and be ready to take the resistance from them, other wise, the increased speed of movement, could be harmful

Ten repetitions are a safe amount. The first several will act as a warm-up for the involved muscles and give the person time to focus and get the feel of the movement.

Use twelve repetitions as the stopping point. In other words, if completing 12 or more reps, in proper style, it is safe to increase the resistance for the next visit.

How much should you increase the resistance? There is no all-inclusive answer to this question. It will require an educated guess. One thing is certain; the resistance increase will be greater than for a standard exercise.

This is due to the negative strength potential of the muscles, much of which may be due to the internal fiber friction. Nevertheless, the potential weight increase can be more than a standard exercise increase.

Complains of muscular soreness are common from those trying this method. This soreness varies, depending on how hard the person worked and the amount of muscle fibers in a particular body segment. The calves, in particular can become so painful, it will be difficult to walk.

This soreness will appear sometime during the day after the exercise, somewhere around the 27th hour mark. Soreness is a companion after each negative exercise program. Not as severe as after the first few visits but, it will always accompany this kind of exercise.

Many people find this soreness very uncomfortable. So, use negative exercise sparingly and allow 4 or more days between visits, to allow for full muscle recuperation. If the pain is unbearable or ads to existing pain, discontinue assisted negative training.

In summary:

> ➤ Negative resistance training requires the help of a qualified supervisor.
> ➤ Muscles are capable of lowering more resistance than they can lift.
> ➤ 40% or more resistance can be lowered than lifted.
> ➤ A controlled speed of movement is recommended. About 10 seconds.
> ➤ Performed only one set of an exercise.
> ➤ Ten repetitions minimum, working to 12 before the resistance is increased.
> ➤ Allow 4 or more days between visits for full recuperation.
> ➤ Do not perform a negative exercise program that includes more than 6 exercises.

Take special not of the speed-of-movement and if it begins to increases' one must know when to stop the movement.

The movement will increase in speed as the muscles tire. When the speed can no longer be termed safe, less than 4 seconds in duration, stop the exercise.

SEQUENCE OF EXERCISE

The sequence of exercises changes each workout. Do not repeat a workout pattern.

Like most interested in strength improvement, you may believe in a structured sequence of exercise. The Sequence of Exercise idea is hereby challenged and put to rest with the tooth fairy myth.

The concept premise is that: "The exercise sequence should be arranged so, the muscles are worked about their relative sizes, from largest to smallest, strongest to weakest."

It further postulates: "In practice, this prescribes that the lower body be worked before the upper body. As a rule, thighs are exercised before the calves, the back, before the chest, and the upper arms before the forearms."

There are at many glaring inconsistencies with those recommendations:

The Most Obvious

- ➤ They are not goal related.
- ➤ Age and possible physical problems are ignored.
- ➤ Genetics is not taken into account.
- ➤ Bodily proportions are disregarded.
- ➤ Target heart rates are misapplied.
- ➤ Muscle strength relationships are not considered.
- ➤ Deteriorating energy levels are over looked.
- ➤ Exercise redundancy is common.
- ➤ Boredom is a common occurrence.
- ➤ Converts to fitness and therapy training become disillusioned.

Each of the examples group under one important call to arms: Goal Directed Exercise. In our terms, it is Rational Exercise.

Let us discuss them as individual portions of a whole.

Goal Directed Exercise

Goal directed exercise is an approach established by analization of one's motive for undertaking fitness training.

Once a goal is established, groups of exercises are selected to achieve the goal, as quickly and safely as possible. Then, a sequence of exercises is selected. The sequence of exercises should relate directly to the goal plan. It is yours and has no relationship to anything other than one's self and individual goals.

Blindly following a sequence recommendation, which someone else uses, is pointless, even if the overall goal is the same. That is because your physical and mental entity is different. This may seem like a minor point. It's not!

Just as an architect constructs a skyscraper starting with a firm foundation, so must a Professional, construct a master plan. That master plan foundation is Goal directed exercise.

First Consideration: The Age Factor

Age influences all actions within Nature. Age, physical and mental problems can limit or enhance an exercise program.

The older a person is, the more care is taken when designing an exercise program. "Everybody knows that," you say. They may, but most health and fitness professionals do not apply the logic of what they know, to an age related program.

As an example: Blood pressure and pulse rates change with age. If an unconditioned older person begins an exercise program by exercising the largest, strongest muscle groups, the blood pressure and pulse rate will rise significantly. Perhaps too much, too soon.

If however, goal related programs began with age, physical and mental condition, as well as previous health profiles in mind, then the program starts by working smaller muscle groups. Ones pulse would not rise considerably.

If you are a rookie and deconditioned person, this might be the approach to take. One may not need to stress the system so much, so soon into the program.

Then, once one is accustomed to exercise, the sequence moves towards the larger muscle groups (if needed). This is a simple example, but I'm sure you get the point.

Sequence of exercise should take into account the age and overall condition of each person. Automatically attacking the largest, strongest area's first, could be the kiss of death. Literally.

Are all 20, 30 or 40 year oldies in the same physical condition? Do they have the exact physical and mental assets or liabilities?

Age by it self, is only one criterion that must be very carefully considered. Present physical condition is another. Beginning an exercise program requires one take age and limitations into account. This is fundamental in any fitness and physical therapy training.

THE ROLE OF GENETICS

Genetics more than anything else, governs your mental and physical potential. Genetics form the origin of our physical universe.

All fitness gains evolve from the Primordial Soup. Genetics more than any other factor, will determine what the sum of our efforts total.

Designing a program without subsequent consideration of one's genetics is irrational at best. It is a waste of time, effort, and money, at worst. Depending on one's genetics, a total body workout may or may not be required.

For example: if one's legs are genetically superior to ones upper body when starting a program, there is no need to be overly concerned about exercising them, unless an injury exists.

Why exercise them at all, until the imbalanced areas develop in proportion to the superior body segments?

Disregarding Bodily Proportions

To disregard genetics is to disregard bodily proportions. In turn, this leads to unbalanced physique development, muscular imbalances, and incomplete fitness levels.

It is impossible for the weaker under developed areas, to catch up with the stronger, better developed body parts, when all areas are worked every workout, to maximum intensity. The advocates of the largest, strongest to smallest, weakest concept, ignore that simple fact.

EXERCISE TARGET HEART RATE

The most popular method of monitoring a trainee's physical status during exercise is by using an estimated
Exercise Target Heart Rate.

In 98% of the gyms we've visited, little attention is given to:

(a) Establishing a reading of the resting pulse rate.
(b) Incorporating a realistic exercise heart rate.
(c) Constant monitoring of the perceived rate.

In our opinion, too much credibility exists to the Heart Rate Chart that relies solely on a person's age and ignores other factors.

Two people of the same age may not be in the same physical condition. Yet, according to the charts, they should begin by working within the same basic target range.

Does that make any sense to you?

Resting heart rate can vary according to age, anxiety, disease, medications, and functional capacity. The charts do not consider these into consideration. If one overlooks these factors, then the base rate will be false.

We have witnessed new clients of fitness centers and therapy clinics, instructed to "warm-up" on a bicycle, until their pulse is within the target heart rate indicated on a chart near the warm-up area.

Setting aside the discussion of exactly what the heart rate should be; there is validity to preparing the heart, alerting it before strenuous exercise.

Whether or not it altering it to the stage of "fight or flight" is safe, is another consideration. To begin an exercise program without properly warming up of the heart can be dangerous, especially if the workout starts with the largest strongest muscle groups and the person if deconditioned.

One cannot establish a person's proper exercise target heart rate by using age as the only limit, any more than one can guess a person's strength level, by asking his or her age. Other factors are important.

Without administering an, in-depth physical history assessment, prior to beginning an exercise program, a proper target heart rate and fitness level, cannot be established.

Guessing at someone's possible reaction to exercise is not good enough. One should know exactly. This can only be achieved with valid, in-depth analization of a person's anatomy, physiology, psyche, and willingness to exercise.

Otherwise, the heart rate charts are almost useless.

MUSCLE STRENGTH RELATIONSHIPS

The strength relationship between muscle groups, on each side of the body and from front to back, must be considered when designing an exercise program.

If for no other reasons than attaining excellent posture and reducing work related fatigue, the strength relationships between muscle groups are important when designing exercise programs.

The largest, strongest crowd never considers this fact. Instead, everyone is instructed to "start here and go there." Always working all basic muscle groups to failure and always following the same sequence.

All we need to do to justify muscle balance is, to observe the posture of many weight trainees or, to observe the posture of those who play one sided sports, such as golf, tennis, and bowling.

Muscle strength relationships relate to all physical aspects of daily life. Imbalance leads to many of life's aches and pains such as: lower back pain, neck and leg pain.

Muscle imbalance can inhibit walking and running gaits. It can cause a golfer to hook or slice a golf ball, and it can affect all sports related performance, as well as on-the-job performance.

In fitness training and physical therapy, one must focus on creating muscular balance. All exercise and therapy programs, which advocate performing exercises with both arms and both legs, against the same lever arm of an exercise machine, are continuing the problem of muscular imbalance.

As are programs using barbells. Dumbbells, used properly, can eliminate muscular imbalance. As will any machine allowing separate movement with each arm or leg.

Muscular balance is often overlooked. Muscular balance for this discussion is, a matching strength, flexibility, and muscular endurance level, between each muscle group, on each side of the body, left to right, front to back.

Muscular balance, in this discussion, does not mean attempting to achieve the exact visual shape to identical muscle groups. For instance, attempting to get the same shape to the right biceps as the left biceps is impossible due to genetic disposition

Muscle shape relates directly to the length of bones, and the origin, insertion and cross-sectional diameter of muscles.

For instance, the biceps strength of the left and right biceps should be in balance with each other, or at least as close. Since origin, insertion and cross-sectional diameter (as well as neuromuscular innervations), relate to the leverage factor of contacting muscles, therefore, it may never be possible, to match muscular strength and muscular endurance on each side of the body.

If it is not possible, a good choice may be to stop trying to strengthen the dominant side muscle groups and focus on the non-dominant sides.

It should not be possible, for example, to curl 40 pounds with the right biceps and only 20 pounds with the left. A clear muscular imbalance exists. This applies to all similar muscle groups and body segments, on each side of the body.

Given the designs of today's equipment and the inherent flaws, just how does one create muscular balance? It's really quite simple.

One must stop using equipment or barbells, which requires two arms or two legs to work against a single lever arm. For example, when one does a leg extension with both legs simultaneously, one is contributing to muscular imbalance one each side of the body.

Although ones functional ability and the exercise resistance may improve, the muscular imbalance between each side will continue, usually in the same proportion as it was at the start of the exercise program.

If one is not using equipment-allowing movement against independent movement\lever arms, one is not doing everything possible to improve balanced performance.

Therefore, one should test for muscular imbalances at the start of the program and work towards eliminating those imbalances.

It is not enough, as is currently supposed, to improve the functional ability by gauging progress on much weight is lifted, without knowing which side is dominant.

As the legs perform a leg extension movement (for example), one leg is contributing more to the movement, than another is.

As the weaker side begins to fail, the stronger side begins to provide a greater percentage of the movement, the weaker side less.

Measure and Improve Imbalances

First, determine the ability to perform, say, the leg extension movement, using two legs at a time.

Then, reduce the resistance to 50 percent of the amount used for the two leg movements. After a short rest, perform as many repetitions as possible with the right leg.

Take a short rest and test the left leg in the same manner.

Here is where you may be surprised.

Many people test better, that is, perform more repetitions, with the so-called non-dominant leg. If a person is right handed therefore thought to be right legged, she or he will accomplish more repetitions with the left leg.

This happens only where repetition movements are performed with a percentage of the one rep maximum resistance.

When one test by first using a one-rep maximum on a single lever machine, then tests for single on rep leg strength, a different imbalance will be discovered.

Apparently, one side can be dominant in strength and the other side dominant in muscular endurance.

All testing is performed in a single side mode. All rehab and fitness programs should take the imbalances in mind, when designing programs.

The approach should be to balance each side with the other.

Accomplish this by first determining which side is non-dominant, in both strength and muscular endurance. Then, continuing to exercise ONLY the non-dominant side, to improve the missing factor.

If you prefer to exercise both sides, then exercise the nondominant side first. Then, the dominant side.

Be sure to stop dominant side movements, at the same amount of repetitions, achieved by the non-dominant side. Otherwise, if repetitions continue with the dominant side the imbalances persist.

Accelerate improvements within a health and fitness program by focusing only on the nondominant issues.

Make adjustments accordingly.

DETERIORATING ENERGY LEVELS DURING EXERCISE

It is obvious that one subtracts from one's fitness level as the exercise program continues; therefore, certain muscles are not properly exercised on a visit to visit basis.

Following the same exercise sequence every visit is the least effective way to enhance total performance.

We know this approach goes against popular opinion. Popular opinion is wrong.

Years ago, we conducted research proving this conclusion. Here's a simple way to think about it: Let's say you have just returned from a restful vacation.

You did nothing physical, had no mental stress, got plenty of sleep and followed a proper diet. You return home completely rested, healthy and looking forward to your workout.

The first thing you notice is that your workout performance is better than during the visit prior to vacation. Even though no workouts are performed during your vacation. You expected your performance would suffer, didn't you?

You performed all your exercises in the usual sequence, and then leave the fitness facility.

Next visit, you do the same sequence and notice you do not feel as good as the last workout and, your performance does not match the last visit. Know why?

You have not fully recuperated between visits. Now, you needed a longer rest time between visits. Not as long as your vacation, but longer than the time between recent visits.

Don't be afraid to learn something about exercise and that is: you need a lot less exercise than you might suppose and more rest than you think.

Physically, this is true. Mentally, you'll often feel as you should stick to your old schedule and exercise more often.

Like most people, you'll probably give into your feelings and get back into the same old rut, even though you learned recuperation improves one's ability to exercise.

We recommend exercising only once every fourth day. This applies to strength training, standard exercise programs, as well as physical therapy programs. Unfortunately, every four days may not fit into your lifestyle.

Now, let us analyze your individual exercise program, to explain why using the same sequence is not as beneficial as mixing up a sequence.

We'll take the best case scenario, the one in which you had just returned from vacation. You walk into the facility and start your exercise sequence. For this illustration, we'll say the program includes 10 exercises.

You do the first exercise. Naturally, since exercise damages the system by making certain biochemical and structural changes, you are no longer as fit as you where before you performed the first exercise. For the sake of easy math, let's say that you damaged your system by 10 percent.

Now, you are going into your second exercise, starting at 90 percent of your best fitness level and you rack up another 10 percent in damages.

Going into your third exercise, you are functioning with 80 percent of the initial 100 percent level. So it goes throughout your total workout.

Since we are making believe that each exercise subtracts 10 percent from your fitness level, by the time you finish the last exercise, number 10, you have depleted 100 percent of your best level.

Because you follow the same sequence during your next visit, you will deplete your reserves in the same manner, for each exercise.

Next visit, by the time you get to exercise #5, you will have depleted 50 percent of your training ability, just as in the last visit. Change the sequence of each exercise, each visit, it allows you to perform different exercises, at a higher level, each visit.

That is to say: if you start with a leg extension on one visit, you apply 100 percent of your ability. If then, you move to the leg curl, you apply 90 percent, etc.

If you reversed the order next visit, then you'd be applying 100 percent on the leg curl and 90 percent on the leg extension, etc.

It's obvious, when one changes a sequence each time, one can exercise some muscles' groups at a higher level than a previous workout. We recommend mixing exercises every visit, to assure maximum progress.

Work weaker muscle group's first, when energy levels are at a higher peak. By nature, most of us prefer to work our best developed, strongest areas.

It makes us feel good, and we usually get favorable comments about our best areas. For maximum progress, we should leave our best areas for later in the program.

This is especially important during physical therapy and functional ability programs. Injured people usually have some associated pain along with the injury. This pain, however slight can reduce one's energy level.

It's best to work the nondominant or the injured area first in a program, before depleting the energy level. Think of the energy level in two ways:

1. The individual body segment energy level. The energy depleted during an exercise of a muscle group. This energy level is somewhat replenished very quickly but not 100 percent. Some depletion takes hours and requires total body sleep to replenish to the 100 percent level.

2. The total body energy. This is the energy that is depleted during exercise of individual body parts. While each body part may replenish itself to a certain level rather quickly, the small percentage not replenished must be rebuilt as indicated in paragraph #1 above.

The apparently small percentages of body segments, energy depletion, total significantly higher that it would appear. That is where total rest is required.

Many times, total recuperation takes several days. The rest days required will vary with the intensity of the exercise program as well as the other stresses of our activities of daily living and work.

The historic exercise treatments of physical disabilities, which ranged from several treatments per day to treatments on a daily basis, have over looked the most important factor of all productive exercise: Rest.

We strongly recommend that you consider approaching strength training, physical therapy, and exercise, from the point of view that rest and the exercise schedule are of equal importance.

For Maximum Results in Minimum Time, combine adequate rest with the following:

(1) Goal directed sequence of exercise.

(2) The muscle strength relationships related to deteriorating energy levels.

(3) Consideration of the age factor.

(4) The role of genetics relating to bodily proportions.

STRENGTH TRAINING BLUEPRINT

THE SIX WEEK PLAN

We are about to outline the step-by-step plan to improve your strength and self-esteem.

It is vitally important that you follow the blueprint exactly as outlined.

You must be ready to accept new guidance and move forward. Do not repeat the mistakes of the past.

We guarantee results if you follow our plan.

THE MASTER PLAN

Total Weekly Workouts. This means you will exercise twice a week with free weights or high-tech equipment, or a combination of both if you wish to.

If possible, exercise every fourth day. This does not mean you cannot walk, swim, play a favorite recreational sport, etc, as often as you want to. We are talking about high-intensity exercise, using high-tech equipment.

If a schedule of every four days is not possible, perform two workouts per week. Workout on a Monday-Thursday, or Tuesday-Thursday schedule.

If that is not possible, pick a sequence of days that allows you at least two-three complete days of rest between workouts.

Remember, if you can handle it emotionally and it fits your lifestyle, workout only every fourth day.

This allows total recuperation between workouts. This every fourth day schedule is our primary recommendation.

Secondarily, we recommend the sequence which allows two-three complete days of rest. The more intensively one exercises, the more rest the body requires between workouts.

With complete recuperation, progress will happen on a workout to workout basis.

GOAL SETTING

Ask yourself, "What is my goal?"

Define your goal and focus on it.

Be prepared to pay the cost in terms of: discipline, persistence, patience and perseverance.

If your goal is to greatly increase your strength, flexibility, muscular endurance, aerobic endurance and reduce your body fat level, have no fear. These are very easy commodities to develop.

In truth all fitness goals are easy to reach once scientific logic and some patience are applied towards them.

If a part of the goal is to reduce your body fat level, then you must combine a low calorie diet with your strength training. To determine how many calories your diet should consume, multiply your present bodyweight by 10. Do not go too far above or below this caloric guideline.

You will not lose muscle tissue as you diet, as long as you are exercising. Muscle tissue loss is common—therefore, a feeling of fatigue and inability to perform daily tasks.

It will take your body about 7—10 days to kick into a weight loss. Be patient. It will happen and your body (and self esteem.) will thank you.

WHAT IS THE MINIMUM AMOUNT OF EXERCISE YOU WILL NEED TO REACH YOUR GOAL?

This is an important question. Remember, the question is not: What is the maximum amount you can perform.

It is, what is the minimum amount needed to reach your goal.

Depending on your knowledge and experience in the exercise arena, you may find it hard to decide how few exercises are actually needed.

Technically, if you exercise at a low intensity, with maximum rest between exercises, you could exercise all day long, to your hearts content.

You will not, however, show any appreciable improvements.

Consequently, if exercise is performed, at a high-intensity level, or performed too often, you cannot exercise for a prolonged period of time.

Exercise done at a maximum level is required for maximum results. The higher level of the intensity you perform, the less you will have to work out.

We recommend twice a week.

GENETIC POTENTIAL AND IT'S MINIMUM AND MAXIMUM EXTREMES

Your genetics (and certain other factors) determine your response to exercise. If for instance, you've inherited a body similar to a female Woody Allen, you will not respond as dramatically to exercise as a body genetically matching model Cathy Ireland or another of that type.

However, all genetic types will respond maximally when a program is scientifically designed.

You already know which are you better developed body areas. You may temporarily ignore these areas when you design a rational fitness program.

It's more important to concentrate on areas that one might term below par, than to continue to over-proportionately develop areas that are already superior. If when designing a rational program you temporarily eliminate those superior areas from your training regimen, you'll benefit in many ways:

- Less total time is spent exercising and more time is allowed for your body to recuperate between workouts. This results in maximum results in minimum time.

- Those areas of your body which were previously lagging will quickly respond to exercise stimulus.

- Unbalanced strength levels, common in virtually all humans, will become more balanced. The net effect being improved physical appearance—more muscular balance and muscular proportion—and, higher energy levels coupled with improved performance in all sports and on-the-job performance.

Obviously, any exercise beyond the minimum required to produce the stimulus for maximum results, is wasted time and energy. Specifically, from the point-of-view of, taxing your recuperative bodily processes.

Remember, improvement cannot take place without adequate bio-chemical rest, and physical and mental recuperation.

Many women use the exercise experience more as a social experience than the athletic performance it is. While this is OK, be advised that you must make up your mind as to whether you want to be a social butterfly or an athlete striving to develop a superior body.

Serious fitness training requires the ability to combine socializing and exercising. Prolonged rambling conversations should be avoided and postponed until a later time.

As we'll indicate in this Blueprint, time is a very important aspect of exercise. There is a difference between actual exercise time and lapsed time.

Exercise time means: the time required to perform each exercise. Elapsed time is the total time of each exercise, plus rest time.

It can be looked at as the time from the start of the program to the program end.

ESTABLISHING YOUR PHYSICAL FITNESS BASELINE

To arrive at a destination you must know where you are starting from and where you are going. Your starting point is your health and fitness Baseline Measurement, including:

- Height, weight, body fat percentage, blood pressure and resting pulse.

- Strength (one repetition maximum).

- Muscular endurance (total reps with a percentage of your one rep maximum) Say—40 %, for the very deconditioned to 80%, for the very fit—of your maximum target heart rate for as many reps as you can perform).

- Aerobic Capacity.

- Flexibility (range-of-motion around a joint).

Any improvement in one aspect is true improvement. One need not improve in each and every area at the same time, every exercise visit; however, if one trains under the proper supervision, it is possible to improve each aspect every visit.

Here's how to establish an exercise baseline to evaluate progress:

If you are presently following an exercise program, pick five exercises from your last workout. A good example would be:

1. Leg Extension, (2. Pulldown (palms toward your face), (3. Bench Press, (4. Overhead Press, and (5. Two Arm Curl.

For these five exercises, multiply the amount of weight used each exercise by the total repetitions you achieved in each. This is you present fitness baseline. You may also record the time of the total exercises.

Follow the advice in this book for six weeks.

At the end of six weeks, it is the time to evaluate your progress. Do this by performing the five exercises used for the baseline measurement and use the same resistance and same sequence as during the baseline test.

This time, exercise to complete muscular failure—defined as: When you can no longer perform a full range repetition in proper form.

Now calculate the improvement percentages.

The improvement between your baseline and your six week evaluation should be startling.

You may choose to retest every six to eight weeks. If so, continue to use a suitable testing baseline. You may continue to use the initial baseline or, if you wish, use the baseline developed during the first six week evaluation.

Progress is slower as your time in the sport increases. In other words, it's harder to become stronger the stronger one becomes.

Continued progress if insured if one stays within the guidelines in this book.

There are so many factors that contribute to and detract from ones progress, it is impossible to guess which is the culprit affecting progress.

Continued progress is always a matter of the process of eliminating negative lifestyle factors. It could range from lack of sleep to over training and poor nutrition.

Life is not easy, contrary to portrayal in the movies or on television.

THE VALUE OF STRENGTH AS COMPARED TO FLEXIBILITY

There can be no progress without a break in tradition. Otherwise, we would still be living in caves, and so it is in the exercise quest. Without challenging tradition, there can be no breakthroughs in any aspect of life.

Many professionals, primarily those in the therapy business, strongly argue that flexibility is more important than strength. Coaches and athletes alike have advanced that same point of view.

We believe strength is of more value than flexibility. We offer the following intellectual ammunition as fact.

Imagine the physical stature of a Woody Allen type body. Put him alongside an Arnold Schwarzenegger type body. Then, picture Woody attempting to twist Arnold's arm at the shoulder to see how flexible Arnold is.

Ask Arnold to do the same to Woody's arm. Whose arm do you think would break and why?

After you accompany Woody down to get his arm in a cast, will you advise him to take more yoga classes or perhaps to tag along with Arnold to the weight room.

The issue of the importance of strength versus flexibility, for preventing injury, has ramifications far beyond hypothetical arm-twisting. Rather, it goes to the heart of fitness training, athletic training, work rehabilitation, physical therapy, and injury prevention.

The American economy loses approximately $40 billion every year because of musculoskeletal back problems alone that damage 80% of the work force.

We use the Woody—Arnold image to illustrate the body's ability to handle complex biomechanical demand, without injury, is usually better served by building adequate and well-balanced strength rather than depending on simply becoming more limber.

Properly conditioned muscles can withstand the long-term stress placed upon them by everyday tasks, and the tremendous amount of sudden impact force. Impact force is simply understood simply as: The weight of an object (your arm, leg, head, or torso), multiplied by the speed of its movement, when pushed, pulled, twisted, or slammed into an object.

When muscles do not absorb the force of your golf swing, overhead tennis smash, or the running gait, the impact transfers to bones.

The predictable, negative results are injury. The flexibility of a yogi will not be able to prevent impact forces from applying torque to a body segment.Back problems are a particular problem for every class of American worker. To understand its sources, we need only visualize the stress we place on the back, almost every minute we are not lying down in a relative stress free position.

Setting all day in your office chair or standing at your counter can be likened to walking around, carrying a five pound object (a dumbbell as an example), which you keep in a perpetual position biceps curl, hands help halfway to shoulder.

Despite the objects, relatively lightness after a while the strain will begin to show. At the end of such a day, you will be reaching for the aspirin (or scotch) bottle, seeking relief.

The back then takes on the muscular stress. It must constantly fight against gravity to hold your torso erect. The effect of a WEAK back commonly appears in the elderly, whose back muscles can no longer support the torso weight erect.

Gravity pulls the torso forward into a stooped position.

A back strengthening program offsets this common problem. With backs and other body segments not meant to handle the upright strain humans put on them daily, any therapy, or rehabilitation protocol without strength as its central focus is doomed to utter failure.

While passive therapies such as, stretching, massage and the like do nothing to improve strengths each has a limited role to play. They do nothing to alter the structural capacity of the muscles to absorb impact stress. Proper strength training will provide adequate structural integrity.

Equally important as muscle strength is muscular balance. This is the relative function and balance of one side of the body compared to the other. This applies in a side to side as well as a back to front plane.

Do not think being an active sports participant will improve the situation. In fact, the opposite is true. Witness the over developed and dominant body segments of golfers, tennis players and bowlers (as examples), it is no accident the display poor posture and have neck, back, shoulder, elbow and wrist problems.

Unfortunately, most of them believe joint pain and poor postures are the cost of sports participation. Lack of strength is the cause not lack of flexibility. The problems compound by well meaning therapists and trainers, who put these athletes on an exercise program without thinking about the problems.

If we agree, for discussion sake, that it is self-evident truth the muscular imbalance exists, and it is caused by one side of the body being dominant than the other, it would make be common sense to design a workout program to focus on NON-DOMINANT areas and ignore the already dominant side.

At least until the weaker areas improve and are in closer relationship to the superior areas. But, nnoooo, instead, programs are designed which exercise both sides, usually with both arms of legs exercising at the same time; Thereby, improving each side, while maintaining the imbalance.

This approach does nothing to improve functional muscular balance between each individual area. Each area improves. The imbalanced ratio stays unchanged. Rather than eliminating the problem, most fitness and therapy programs continue on the right track but heading in the wrong direction.

High-Tech exercise machines and new concepts of exercise allow one to achieve maximum fitness in minimum time; however, proper use of this equipment and application of new techniques to improve fitness and functional abilities remain ignored by many.

Instead, they continue the dogma of the past. Never thinking about or accepting a new, improved approach. Myths, misconceptions, oldwife's tales, and outright lies prevail and everyone loses.

Dedicating more thought and time to proper strength training reduces or eliminates work injuries, daily activity injuries, and sports related injuries.
It is time to introduce sane thinking into the present approach to health and fitness exercise and physical therapy.

BODY STRUCTURE
DOMINANT AND NON-DOMINANT CONSIDERATIONS

You goal is to improve you total body balance by improving the elements of body balance between the right and left sides of your body, to within 10 percent of each other.

We have previously outlined The Life Force Index and explained how to find your one repetition maximum strength and your muscle endurance. You follow a similar approach to test for the dominant and non-dominant structures.

Use the same five exercises and the same testing approach. The only difference is this test is done in a one arm or one leg fashion. The exercises to use are:

1. Leg Extension
2. Bench Press
3. Pull-down to chest, from overhead, palms towards the face.
4. Overhead Press.
5. Two Arm Curl.

Initially you performed these using two arms or two legs. This time you will follow the advice of as an alternative, using one leg or one-arm movements.

First, testing for your one repetition maximum. Then, you use a percentage of the maximum attempt to determine your maximum muscle endurance.

Follow this procedure:

1. Begin with the leg extension. Choose an amount of light resistance to use with your dominant leg, and warm up the muscles and joints for a one-minute continuous movement.

(a) Then, add a small increase in weight and perform only one repetition and, increase the weight slightly to perform another one repetition with your dominant leg. Continue this sequencing until you reach your one repetition maximum lift.

(b) After you establish your one rep maximum strength level, the next step is to determine your muscle endurance with a percentage of your max weight.

Choose between 50 percent up to 80 percent for this test. After a short rest, load the amount of resistance you will use for the test and perform as many controlled, full range repetitions as you can.

(c) Now, you have determined the strength and muscular endurance of your dominant leg. Write that information down on your chart and get ready to test the non-dominant leg in the same way.

Testing your non-dominant leg exactly follow the procedure in paragraph 1, and subparagraphs a, b, and c as written above.

Be sure to use the same percentage of the maximum one repetition resistance with the non-dominant as you did with your dominant leg. Do not be surprised if you perform more repetitions with you non-dominant leg. This leg may test weaker in strength but it will test higher in endurance.

We believe: The so-called non-dominant body segment rests on a day-to-day basis, because the dominant side does more work during the day.

It appears that rested muscles are more capable of producing more prolonged work than muscles, which are partially fatigued.

Retain the valuable data for future reference. You will be vastly surprised when a retest is given and you experience the results.

We will share one great training method you might employ, which, as many concepts we share with you, seem contradictory to your present knowledge base. At least until you experience the truth of our research.

Training for, and attaining body balance requires a different dedication and approach to exercise than used in a standard workout approach.

It demands the discipline to only exercise the present non-dominant elements towards improvement, and to exercise the dominant parts in a way that seeks only to maintain the present fitness level, making no effort to improve them.

Here is what that would look like when following a Life Force Body Balance Program©. This procedure directly relates to the baseline data you generated, when you tested each body area, in an individual way and arrived at a one-rep maximum and a maximum muscle endurance level.

This approach determined the true dominant, non-dominant elements of strength and muscle endurance of each area; however, the dominant strength may be (as an example) on the right side and the dominant endurance may be on the left side (as an example).

Your initial data may look something like the following example of the leg extension data:

One Rep Max		Muscle Endurance with 70% of Max
Right side:	100 lbs.	14 repetitions
Left side:	60 lbs.	21 repetitions

This data indicates that the right side is 100 strong and develops 14 repetitions of muscle endurance. The left side is only 60 strong (40% less than the right side) and produces 21 repetitions (7 reps more endurance) than the right side.

Self-evident truth in this example is the strength dominant right side. Exercise this side to produce more muscle endurance and not more strength—until the left side strength closes the gap, and becomes stronger in relation to the right side.

It is also clear that; the non-dominant left side muscle endurance is superior to the muscle endurance of the right side and is not a problem at this point.

We say "no problem" because as you train to improve the strength level of the left side, following the Life Force protocol, the muscle endurance gains will be in balance to the strength gains. Eventually, as you balance both sides of the body, and begin to exercise body sides together, all strength and muscle endurance gains coexist together.

Your program design, using the above example, would be to determine an amount of weight to use on all strength dominant side that allows 15 repetitions. Stay with that resistance and that amount of repetitions.

If you use more weight, even though you probably could, you will increase the dominance. As areas balance out begin to increase the resistance. This is a temporary body-balancing attempt.

Left side exercises are exactly as indicated in the Chapter 22 outline of The Life Force Index, increasing the resistance at the right time. Before long, in about one month, both sides closely balance. Then, you begin to work both sides for maximum increases.

The genesis of this approach is proper training for strength increases will, at the same time, increase the muscle endurance level. The opposite is not true, one cannot train to increase endurance and have strength increase at the same time. That is just the way the human body functions.

We have often tested the strength and endurance levels of long distant runners who dislike strength training. They continue to exercise only to increase cardio endurance.
When we retest them months (sometimes years) later, there is no increase in strength levels. In fact, they are usually weaker than during the previous test. This has proven to be true in all cases.

Finally, after following these procedures, for one month, conduct a retest in exactly the manner you did to compile your baseline data. If everything tests out to only a 10 percent difference between body parts, it is OK to begin training in the standard way.

Actually, here is the kicker. For continued maximum gains and to insure muscular balance, you should continue an exercise program in which you exercise each side of the body independently of each other.

This would mean you should continue to do exercises allowing each side to lift a certain amount of resistance, independent or the other side helping with the attempt.

In the next chapter, we will outline that approach in detail.

ALTERING BODY STRUCTURE

We have previously mentioned that body structure is genetic. All body structures will improve beyond "normally" acquired strength, flexibility, and muscular endurance and cardio endurance.

A major flaw of most of the high-tech fitness equipment in the marketplace is: The equipment is not designed to allow individual movements of opposite sides of the body, meaning: Most movements are produced by produced by either arm or legs producing the movement.

Technically, this is movement produced by a single level arm. The single lever arm is the part of the machine you would push or pull against to lift the resistance.

As an example, when seated in a leg extension machine and you push forward to lift the resistance both legs are pushing against the padding that is part of the single lever arm and both the dominant and non-dominant legs (as described in the previous chapter) are lifting the weight.

The exercise is more effective when lifting the resistance with independent movements, individually produced with each leg.

If the exercise equipment you have access to be the type mentioned above, it is possible to change the function to your advantage. All you need do is adjust the resistance so you are exercising only one leg to fatigue. Then, exercise the opposite leg to fatigue. That is counted as one set.

This technique is the most productive for body balance and overall gains. The only drawback—it will double your workout time. A small price to pay for greater results!

If you prefer, you could use dumbbells for most of your workout. Dumbbells, as we explained in Chapter 20, are not as productive as high-tech equipment; however, they will produce better body balance than using either barbells (single lever arm) or machines that require use of single lever arms.

Any exercise program designed to allow independent movements of separate body segments is superior to those demanding combined arm or leg movements.

Arguably, single arm of single leg movements will reduce the cardio benefit but by how much relates to the personal fitness level of the trainee.

The use of one arm or one leg at a time is also less invasive and less stressful to the system than using two arms or two legs at the same time. Although the law of Force-Counter Force is still valid, the amount of resistance is much less and in more proportion to the body structure.

Give thought to changing the perception that "weight must feel heavy" in order to be beneficial. It does not have to feel heavy; it just has to allow you to exercise the muscles in a safe, controlled manner until the muscle fatigues.

CREATING THE FIRST WORKOUT

This chapter speaks in a way outlining a proper professional discussion between a client (you), AND as a Private Fitness Trainer, Physical Therapist, or Work Rehabilitation Professional should outline your program for you

This method is part of our Life Force protocol for professionals, and is adapted from our book "Life Force Fitness Therapy." We created this approach 30 years ago and have used it successfully in the environments of fitness centers, physical therapy facilities, hospitals, medical centers, chiropractic offices, and work rehabilitation sites.

We believe this two-fold discussion between the professional and the client will help you understand, both the role the therapist should play, and the role you can play in formulating your success.

In addition, we feel this dual interview-overview will present you with basic knowledge you may use to assist a family member or friend, undertake a safe, effective exercise program.

Get ready to put on your acting attitude and play both parts in the fitness chapter of your life.

Any words written in this typeface are you acting and talking as a Life Force Fitness Therapy Professional.

This typeface is the author talking as the professional.

Get ready, the show lights are darkening, the audience is quieting, the music swells and...YOU ARE ON STAGE;

The opening scene is the author talking to the professional and saying....

You have listened to the client's complaints, injuries, issues, wishes, and wants. Begin to reassure her that lack of results is typical, given the typical approach to fitness.

Professionals explain that: In order to really reach goals she must first establish "Where she is in a physical sense". Mention that no other fitness centers do it in the way you do, and you have schooled in the Life Force concept. This means evaluate to establish her **Life Force Index.**

You might say something like this: *"Katherine, in order to design a wellness program the first thing we must do is collect accurate information—in a safe and specific way—about your <u>present</u> <u>physical</u> <u>condition</u>. In simple terms, this means your present levels of strength, flexibility, and endurance.*

Once we establish your present baseline, we will know the fastest, safest path to your goals. No one should be accepted into an exercise program without first determining the baseline Fitness Index in a way that is safe, effective and within your personal abilities.

We are not going to force you to exercise beyond your ability or compare you with any-one else. We are interested in focusing our attention on you and having you, focus attention on yourself and that is what we will do.

Katherine, what we are about to do is this: You are going to perform—in a safe way— a series of only 5 exercises that will tell us your fitness level. Chances are your fitness level is better than you think it is. So, do not be concerned about not doing well. You will do fine. Five exercises do not seem like many but it will be more work than it sounds like, and it will take about one half hour.

During the testing, <u>I</u> <u>will</u> <u>not</u> <u>encourage</u> <u>or</u> <u>discourage</u> <u>you</u> <u>in</u> <u>any</u> <u>way</u>; or force you to do anything more or less, than you feel like doing. I want you determine how much effort you want to put into the testing. You do not have to prove you are superwoman to me and I am not going to attempt to prove I can work you to exhaustion. You just to the very best you can."

This statement gives permission to fail and allows the client to feel OK if they have set false impressions of what they should achieve.

By now, the client should be feeling confident and comfortable given the reassur-ances you have presented. Hearing the word <u>safe</u> several times and emphasizing everything are associated with her wishes and goals will eliminate the fear of "being worse than others".

Katherine, does everything make a sense so far?"

You now continue to briefly explain the test by discussing the 5-exercise protocol.

THE FIVE-EXERCISE PROTOCOL

While still in your office you continue by saying: *"Katherine, beginning with the first exercise you will determine your strength level. We will do it in the following way.*

- *First, we will adjust the machine so you are comfortable and properly aligned (assuming you are using a machine).*

- *Then, we will take a light weight and you will do the movement for about one minute. This is a warm up for the muscles and the joints involved in the motion. This indicates your range-of-motion or flexibility measurements that we follow.*

- *Once you have warmed up, I am going to pick a certain amount of weight that I know is safe for you and I want you to start a series of <u>one repetition movement</u>. Even though it may feel light, you just do one movement. Then stop the movement.*

- *Then, I am going to make the weight a little bit heavier and you do one more and stop. What we are doing Katherine, is to continue making the weight a little bit heavier for every repetition. After a while, you will notice the resistance feeling heavier. That is a signal from your body that it hasn't felt anything like this and it is also a safe signal the body sends to get your attention that you are in the safe zone, capable of more, if you feel OK about doing more.*

- *Katherine, when you start feeling this signal you may feel anxious that maybe you do not want to lift more. It is OK to stop. So just let me know and we can stop. All it means is that you have reached your mental or physical limit on that exercise.*

- *If you feel comfortable trying more we will continue, until you feel you have done your best.*

Now it is time to move to the exercise area and begin the test.

Author's note: It is of <u>crucial</u> <u>importance</u> that once the baseline strength levels are established no other maximum one rep strength session be attempted until AFTER the first 30 day exercise period.

STRENGTH TESTING AND THE ONE REPETITION MAXIMUM

Remember the five exercises you will use are: (1) Leg Extension, (2) Bench Press, (3) Pullover or Pull down in front, (4) Overhead Press and (5) Two Arm Curls. It is important to use this sequence, so in a busy facility, just try to time it so that this approach is possible.

The Warm Up

➢ Move to the leg extension machine and use whatever method you use to demonstrate the proper form. To effectively manage time, we <u>do not sit</u> on the machine, we prefer to pull the weight pins and guide the clients onto the machine, ask her to perform a few controlled movements throughout her comfortable range-of-motion.

When you are satisfied with the performance, end the demonstration. Choose a proper warm up weight to use for 60 seconds. When you have the weight set, the client begins the movement, and you step out of the direct sight of the client.

➢ Step slightly behind her and at the area slightly behind the shoulder. This position allows you to supervise and allows the client to concentrate on performance. Once the minute warm up is finished step forward into the line of sight and tell her to stop the movement.

The Strength Test

The client's leg muscles are warmed up, and it is time to choose a starting, one repetition weight for the leg extension.

Remember—after the first repetition—increase in about two and one half pound or five pound increments. Increase before each repetition, as the weight stack moves down and touches together at the bottom of the movement. If you pick the proper starting weight for the one repetition movement, it will not take long to reach muscular failure, about 10 single repetition movements.

➢ Decide on a safe amount of weight to perform one repetition with and give the following instructions to the client.

➢ *"Katherine, what we're going to do now is a series of one repetition movement. I am going to pick a weight that I would like you to do only one repetition with and then I want you to stop the movement. I will increase the weight slightly and then I will ask you to do another repetition and stop the movement. We will continue that sequence: You do a repetition and I will increase the weight etc. We are safely, slowly working towards your maximum strength level.*

> *As we approach your maximum strength level, you will receive a signal from your brain that the weight is beginning to feel heavy. The signal is a safe sign that you are safely within your strength level and that it is OK to continue if you are comfortable with lifting more weight. At that point, you can choose to continue or not. You tell me what you would like to do."*

If the client stops upon the first sign of the resistance feeling heavy, so be it.

Many times, muscular pain related to the leg muscles are severe to an untrained individual and may account for her not being able to continue. If she chooses to continue, do so until muscular failure occurs. Chart the result on the workout card. Give the client a slight rest appropriate to her effort. Then, advance to the Endurance Test (If you've decided to perform both tests on the same day).

THE MUSCLE ENDURANCE TEST

If you make the decision that this person is capable of completing both the strength test and the endurance test during this visit, it is time to begin the data gathering for both baselines.

First, rate the leg extension for a maximum repetition attempt with a certain percentage of the maximum strength level. If the decision is to perform the endurance test on another day, move on to the bench press for the Strength Test assessment.

Combining both tests during the same visit is safe and vigorous. It is also a total effort. Test results are accurate if you do both tests together or on separate days. We prefer to do both tests on the same day.

The deconditioned will require more rest between the one rep maximum attempt and the maximum repetition attempt. It is may be a better idea to reschedule the endurance test for the next visit for some injured, deconditioned people.

A word of caution: Do not include any other physical exercise on the same day as these tests. Just do the baseline data gathering.

If the decision is to go for the endurance test allow the client a minute or so rest and continue after choosing a percentage of the maximum, one repetition lifts for the endurance test.

Assume the client has reached a point of failure with 100 lbs. and cannot do another repetition in proper form. You now know the exact one repetition strength of that body segment on that day. It is time to offer congratulations with a—*"That was well done!"* Say <u>something</u> in a positive way.

If you have made the decision to also test this client for muscular endurance, it is time to explain the next step.

First, check to make sure everything is OK. Ask if she wants some water or a short time-out. Then proceed.

"Katherine that was really well done. Now that we know your strength level, we will test for muscle endurance. Here is how we will do that.

- *I am going to take an amount of weight that is <u>less than</u> what you just lifted, so it will feel lighter to you. What I would like you to do is to do as many repetitions as you can.*
- *Remember Katherine, I am not going to encourage or discourage you, and I want you to decide how many you can do. Whatever that amount is, it will be fine with me. Do the best you can. OK, are you ready to go? Just be sure to control the movement in a safe manner. Start when you are ready."*

When testing for <u>muscular endurance,</u> most women feel physically and emotionally comfortable with a weight that feels light rather than heavy. Most men prefer the feel of "heavier" weight physically and emotionally.

As an example: 60% to 70% "feels" like enough to a woman. 80% would be a maximum we would recommend. More than 80% will greatly reduce the performance for all other than the very strong and most highly motivated.

For many men, 80% of the one repetition maximum work well with all exercises. You may have to use a lower percentage based on what you know about the client. Use a common sense. There is nothing magic about using any <u>certain percentage</u> of the maximum lift.

Regardless of the percentage used, the data will be accurate for that person. In one month, when the retest is given, you will be able to compare the initial data with retest data.

The percentages we have used relate to the brand name of equipment we prefer. We prefer MedX and Nautilus. The point we are making is that dissimilar equipment produce different "feels".

This is because of the design and inherent friction components. Therefore, 80% on a MedX machine would feel very comfortable and on another design may feel like a "ton". Use your discretion but establish consistent percentages to use with each person, related to their psyche and genetics.

Now, back to *Katherine*

As she performs the movement, watch the body position, speed-of-movement, pausing between repetitions and so on. If she strays from acceptable form, step into her line of sight and offer a brief statement, such as *"A little slower as you are lifting the weight... That's fine!"* Then, step back out of the direct line of sight, a little behind the shoulders. The idea is to let her concentrate without eye-to-eye contact or by feeling intimidated.

When she completes her best attempt, she will automatically stop. At that point, step back into her vision and congratulate her on a well-done performance.

Chart the data, including the seat position, use of any back pads, range of motion, etc. Keep an eye on the clock. Do not get trapped into a long explanation of useless information. A minute to a minute and one half is usually enough time for most people to recover. If you feel more time is required, do so.

Tell her some positive things you have observed about her performance. Then move on to the second exercise, the bench press.

Remember to use the sequence we have described, if this equipment is available or substitute similar equipment for the related muscle groups.

1. Leg Extension
2. Bench Press
3. Pullovers or Pull down in Front
4. Overhead Press
5. Two Arm Curl

Obviously, if the person has an injury that prohibits a certain exercise, use your knowledge base to substitute one that is appropriate.

THE SECOND EXERCISE AND BEYOND

Beginning with the second exercise and continuing through to the fifth exercise, everything becomes easier. The client has an idea of what is required for her to produce valid data and you have an idea of her ability to concentrate and perform according to your instructions.

We recommended the following points for the remaining exercises:

As you get ready for the bench press exercise, adjust the machine for the right body positioning, etc.:

❖ Offer a brief overview of what is about to take place: (1) The one-minute warm-up followed by (2) The one repetition movement to failure, (3) A brief rest and (4) Using a percentage of the maximum to test muscular endurance.

❖ Start the strength test with a reasonable resistance. Do not attempt to begin too heavy and do not attempt large weight increases.

❖ It is difficult to recommend to you exactly how much to increase the resistance between repetitions during the strength test. It varies depending on the genetic potential of the client. One may have large, strong leg muscles and smaller weak biceps muscles. The increases would vary accordingly. When in doubt use smaller weight increments rather than larger and use the common sense approach.

❖ You will know you are in the ballpark if your client fails within about ten repetitions during the strength test.

You will find that some exercises require assistance. As an example:

➤ A bench press machine, a pullover machine, or a pull down movement may require that you hand (or pull) the bar moving the weight into position during the start of every strength testing repetition—after you have reloaded and increased the resistance. All you need do is get the bar into the client's hands and very slowly release after you ask them if they have a grip.

➢ Then, after they perform one rep you take the bar from them, reload, and hand it back to them. It is OK if these "reload and hand back to the client" takes 10 to 15 seconds. Just try to keep a consistent time between repetitions. Do not take 15 seconds at one time and are led into talking for 60 seconds or more during other reloading procedures. Be consistent!

Follow the same exact sequencing as during the first exercise. Follow the sequence, chart the data, allow adequate rest, and verbally reward the client after each exercise.

How to Lose Weight Quickly and Safely

"I eat like a bird, why do I gain weight?" Every time someone says that to you, ask:" What kind of bird—a sparrow or a vulture?"

Studies have shown there is a direct correlation between a people being inactive and weight gain. Experts say it is inactivity, not necessarily excess eating that can add excess body fat. Misinformation contributes to unhealthy dieting practices.

For instance—we recently talked with a woman who was following a well known franchised diet plan. Her diet consultant recommended she should not exercise while dieting. That advice is pure and simple hogwash!

Quite the opposite is true. Medical journals have indicated one will lose muscle tissue when dieting, unless you exercise program at the same time. The exercise approach will retain and contribute to an increase in lean tissue.

Muscle tissue is productive tissue, that is: muscles provide human movement. Therefore, any loss of productive muscle tissue lends itself to a loss of high level function in daily activities.

Weight loss and weight control requires four closely interrelated functions: (1) diet, (2) exercise, (3) behavioral modification and (4) a support system. One must have each of these in place to experience healthy weight loss.

Diet

Intake of less than 1200 calories on a daily basis is generally discouraged. Unless one is under physician supervision. 1200 calories can provide the body with enough energy and nourishment to allow bodily functions to take place.

Calories should be supplied in a certain ration of protein to fat and carbohydrate. Most research indicates fats be kept to a minimum, carbohydrates should be eaten in the highest proportion and proteins eaten at about a medium level. As one example: 75% carbohydrate, 15% protein and 10% fat.

These recommendations vary slightly from research study to research study. For safety sake, check with your physician or other knowledgeable professional before undertaking any diet or exercise program.

A healthy diet should:

1. Satisfy all nutrient needs.
2. Be acceptable to individual tastes and habits.
3. Minimize hunger and eliminate fatigue.
4. Be readily available and socially acceptable.
5. Favor establishment of a lasting pattern of eating.
6. Be conductive to improvement of overall health habits.

Combined with a healthy low calorie diet, exercise produces the flame to ignite the weight loss process.

Exercise

The following exercise recommended guidelines can produce excellent results for dieter's.

1. Frequency: Three to five days per week. The higher the intensity of exercise—high tech—under supervision requires only two workouts per week. Low intensity exercise can be followed on a daily basis (walking, etc.)
2. Intensity: 60% of ones maximum heart rate.
3. Duration: 30 minutes to 45 minutes.
4. Type of activity: Any activity using large muscle groups, in rhythmic movement. Examples: walking, jogging, swimming, cycling or any endurance type game or activity and of course high-tech exercise.

Behavioral Modification & Support

Behavior modification is the most difficult to master and most complex of the components. Here are some guidelines that work:

1. Keep accurate records on a daily basis.
2. Eat foods you enjoy but know when to stop.
3. Enlist the support of friends and relatives.
4. Weigh yourself once a day—morning is best.

5. Don't expect to lose more than two to three pounds of fat per week. Three pounds is a LOT of fat. Next time you are at a meat counter, ask the butcher for three pounds of fat. Seeing is believing.

7. Expect about a seven to ten day lag time before your diet kicks in and your weight begins to drop. Don't give up too soon.

8. Divide your total calories into many small meals, instead of three large meals.

9. Eat most of the calories prior to 4 PM. No snacking at night.

10. Set realistic long term goals. Be patient. You can do it.

Staying healthy and fit is a way of life. It requires above average discipline, motivation, and patience.

Everyone making the commitment to lose excess body fat and becomes fit agrees: Once you achieve wellness, you will never want to be average again.

You can and should do it.

Go for it!

A Sample 1200 Calorie Diet

The following recommendations are those serving choices allowed in each column. Select any of the servings listed in each column but, do not exceed the recommended serving amounts.

This will appear to be a LOT of food; however, this diet provides adequate energy to prevent fatigue and provides one with a feeling that eliminates the urge to snack between meals.

3 servings per day

Skim milk or skim milk yogurt (omit one daily fat serving for each serving if you use low fat milk) (omit two daily fat servings for each serving if you use whole milk)

3 servings per day

1 oz. cold cuts
1 oz. Hamburg (omit 1 fat serving)
1 oz. cheddar cheese (omit 1 fat serving)
1 oz. Lean beef, pork, veal, lamb, fish, or poultry (no skin)
1/4 c. cottage cheese
1/2 c. Beans or peas with 1 bread serving
2 tsp. Peanut butter (omit 2 daily fat servings if this is chosen)

6 servings per day

1/2 c. unsweetened cold cereal, rice, pasta, cooked cereal
3 c. popcorn
6 saltine crackers
3 rye wafers
4 soda crackers
1/2 c. beans or peas
1 slice bread 1/2 bagel or English muffin
15" pancake or waffle (omit 1 daily fat serving)

1/2 c. winter or acorn squash
1/4c. Yams

4 servings per day

Fats—omit any servings used in other groups
1 tsp. margarine
1 tsp. butter
1 tsp. oil
1 tsp. Lard
1 tsp. mayonnaise
1 strip of bacon
2 tsp. Sour cream
2 tsp. Light cream
1 tsp. French or Italian dressing
1 tbsp. cream cheese
1 tbsp. heavy cream
20 Spanish peanuts
10 almonds
2 whole pecans
10 peanuts
6 walnuts
6 other nuts

2 servings per day

1/2 cup of:

Asparagus bean sprouts
Broccoli
Brussels sprouts
Cabbage
Carrots
Cauliflower
Celery
Eggplant
Green pepper
Greens mushrooms
Okra
Onions

String beans
Summer squash
Tomatoes
Tomato juice
Turnip
Zucchini

5 servings per day

Small apple
1/2 c. unsweetened applesauce
2 fresh apricots
1/2 grapefruit
1/4 C. grape juice
1/4 cantaloupe
1 c. watermelon
1 orange
1 peach
1/2 c. apple juice
1/2 small banana
4 dried apricots
1/2 c. berries
3/4 C. strawberries
12 grapes
1/8 honeydew
1 nectarine
1/2 C. orange juice
1 pear
1/2 C. pineapple
2 plums
2 tbsp. raisins
1/3 C. pineapple juice
2 prunes
1 tangerine

This illustration of a 1200 calorie diet is included in this book as one example of many you may choose to follow.

We again recommend you check with your physician prior to starting any exercise or diet program.

CALORIES EXPENDED IN VARIOUS PHYSICAL ACTIVITIES

Following are examples of the various calories used to perform certain tasks. They are listed in a calories per minute basis.

To determine the amount of calories one "burns" during the course of daily activities, all one need do is multiply the calorie per minute number by the amount of minutes one performs that activity.

You will be surprised at how little energy one actually uses's up during the course of daily activities.

To lose body fat, one must burn more calories during the course of the day than one consumes.

Calories Expended in Various Physical Activities

ACTIVITY	CAL/MIN
Ping Pong—Table Tennis	4.9-7.0
Calisthenics	5.0
Rowing: Pleasure—Vigorous	5-15
Cycling: 515 MPH (10 speed)	5-12
Skating: Recreational—Vigorous	5-15
Archery	5.2
Badminton: Recreational—Competitive	5.-10
Basketball: Half Full Court	6-9
(More for fast break)	
Bowling (while active)	7.0
Tennis: Recreational—Competitive	7-11
Water Skiing	8.0
Soccer	9.0
Snow shoeing (2.5 MPH)	9.0

Handball and Squash	10.0
Mountain Climbing	10.0
Judo and Karate	13.0
Football (while active)	13.3
Wrestling	14.4

Skiing:

Moderate to Steep	8-12
Downhill Racing	16.5
Cross Country: 3-8 MPH	9-17

Swimming:

Pleasure	6.0
Crawl: 2550 yds/min	6-12.5
Butterfly: 50 yds/min	14.0
Backstroke: 2550 yds/min	6-12.5
Breast stroke: 2550 yds/min	6-12.5
Side stroke: 40 yds/min	11.0

Dancing:

Modern: Moderate—Vigorous	4.2-5.7
Ballroom: Waltz—Rumba	5-7.0
Square	7.7

Walking:

Road or Field (3.5 MPH)	5—7.0
Snow: Hard\Soft (3.52.5 MPH)	10-20
Uphill: (3.5 MPH)	8-11-15
Downhill: (2.5 MPH)	3-3.5
1520% (2.5 MPH)	3.7-4.3
Hiking: 40 lb. pack (3.0 MPH)	6.8

Running:

12 min. mile (5 MPH)	10
8 min. mile (7.5 MPH)	15
6 min. mile (10 MPH)	20
5 min. mile (12 MPH)	25

Standing, light activity	2.6
Washing and dressing	2.6
Washing and shaving	2.6
Driving a car	3.1
Washing clothes	3.1
Walking indoors	3. 1
Shining shoes	3.2
Making bed	3.4
Dressing	3.4
Showering	3.4
Cleaning windows	3.8
Carpentry	3.8
Farming chores	3.8
Sweeping floors	3 9
Plastering walls	4.1
Truck and automobile repair	4.2
Ironing clothes	4.2
Farming, planting, hoeing, raking	4.7
Mixing cement	4.7
Mopping floors	4.9
Repaving roads	5.0
Gardening, weeding	5.6
Stacking lumber	5.8
Stone, masonry	6.3
Pick and shovel work	6.7
Farming, haying, plowing with horse	6.7
Shoveling (miners)	6.8
Walking downstairs	7.1
Chopping wood	7.5
Gardening, digging	8.6
Walking upstairs	10-18
Pool or billiards	1.8
Canoeing: 2.54.0 MPH	3.0-7.0
Volleyball: Recreational—Competitive	3.5-8.0
Golf: Foursome—Twosome	3.7-5.0
Horseshoes	3.8
Baseball (except pitcher)	4.7

A Final Note

A final note: We believe there are many benefits one can derive from rational exercise some known, others yet unknown. We offer the following article by Jane E. Brody of the New York Times as a recent discovery that benefits women.

Is there a possibility that exercise may also benefit men in the sense of preventing some kinds of cancers?

Exercise Found To Cut Risk of Breast Cancer

A new study of more than 1,000 California women has found that moderate but regular physical activity can reduce a woman's risk of developing pre-menopausal breast cancer by as much as 60 percent.

The benefits were greatest among women who had borne children and those who were physically active in their teenage years and early 20s.

The most striking reduction in risk was found among women who exercised for four hours a week, doing activities like jogging, swimming laps or playing tennis. But even as few as two to three hours of weekly exercise was beneficial, reported Dr. Leslie Bernstein, who directed the study.

The results are described in today's issue of The Journal of the National Cancer Institute by Bernstein and her colleagues at the University of Southern California's North Cancer Center.

If confirmed by further studies, the finding, which at the moment applies only to women 40 years or younger, singles out exercise as the first risk factor for breast cancer that women can readily control.

"This could be an extremely important finding," said Dr. Lynn Rosenberg, an epidemiologist at the Boston University School of Medicine. "There's not any method at the moment that women could practically use to reduce their risk of getting breast cancer."

In an editorial accompanying the study, Dr. Louise Brinton of the National Cancer Institute said the new finding was especially important because it seemed to identify exercise as an independent factor influencing the risk of breast cancer.

Dr. Rosenberg commented that "even if the results are not con firmed, there are a thousand other reasons that women should exercise." Among other things, regular exercise reduces a woman's chances of developing heart disease, osteoporosis, diabetes and hypertension.

Other established risk factors for breast cancer include family history, age at menarche, age at first pregnancy, number of pregnancies and socioeconomic status.

Risk is lowest among those who start menstruating late, who have their first child by the age of 20 and who have a greater number of pregnancies. There may also be some protective effect from breast feeding.

All these factors are associated with a diminished release of the ovarian hormones estradiol and progesterone, which appear to
Influence the development or growth of breast cancer.

Although various dietary factors have been proposed as influencing the risk of breast cancer, none have been firmly established.

In the new study, lifetime exercise habits and other relevant factors were determined through interviews with 545 women 40 years and younger with newly diagnosed breast cancer and an equal number of women free of cancer but otherwise comparable.

Dr. Bernstein said in an interview that there were still many unanswered questions. Among them, she said, are when in life women must exercise to be protected and whether breast cancer in post menopausal women might also be reduced by physical activity.

Although the study shows that physical activity in adolescence and early adulthood had the greatest benefit, Dr. Bernstein said, "We still saw a very strong protective effect among the women who became active later on."

The Final View

The previous chapter outlines the basics of designing a fitness, physical therapy, or work performance program.

Once the baseline data is determined, future workouts are designed from the baseline. There are so many combinations of exercises one may use in a wellness program, it is impossible to list them in this book. My advice is to purchase a book that instructs and illustrates the proper form of exercise performance.

For now, all one must do is visit a local bookstore, library or magazine stand to find information on various exercises.

As long as you follow the information in this book or other products we produced, your progress is guaranteed.

If you have any questions or need our personal guidance with your programs feel free to contact us at: safe-life@worldnet.att.net and we will be happy to help.

THANK YOU FOR YOUR SUPPORT!

As the creator of this book and others, I want to thank you for the kindness you express by purchasing this product.

I offer it to you with the intent of teaching you many valuable ideas to help you improve your lifestyle and wellness.

May the Source be with you!

Joseph F. Mullen

AFTER SIX WEEKS AND BEYOND

The guidelines in this book are valid and applicable into eternity (so to speak). Unfortunately, exercise becomes very boring for most people.

It therefore becomes necessary to find ways of altering an exercise approach. In practice this requires variety in exercise.

Listing the myriad of possible exercises is beyond the space available for this book. Suffice it to say variety is good and should be considered safe and productive.

We recommend one vary exercises as often as needed. Exercise can be fun.

There is nothing (within reason) you cannot accomplish with motivation, discipline and devotion to your cause; however, it will require hard work.

We believe you are of the right stuff to apply yourself to a goal and to stick to it.

FOR MORE INFORMATION

For more information about Books, Audio Tapes, CDs and Consultations by Joseph Mullen, contact him at: safe-life@worldnet.att.net

<u>The Fitness Center Owner's Manual</u> ©: *How to Succeed in the fitness business.*

If you are presently in the fitness or physical therapy business or ever dreamed of having, a facility of your own this is the book for you. It contains comprehensive, "How to" information combined with decades of personal experience and proven advice related to business survival.

<u>The Fitness Instructor Manual</u> ©: *Everything you need to know for employment, full or part-time as a respected Fitness Instructor.*

Covers all aspects from "How to" become a Fitness Instructor to designing safe, fitness and therapy protocols to produce maximum results in minimum time. A foolproof approach to financial health.

<u>The Ultimate Workout Journal</u> ©

Initially conceived, for purchase only by fitness center owners to sell to clients or to use as a sales incentive. It contains answers to basic fitness related knowledge most consumers' lack. It is now available to consumers and professionals.

<u>Secret's of Advanced Nautilus Training</u> ©

This concise information is available in Book form or as *a two hour, audiocassette and CD.*

It contains new approaches to exercise as well as the comparisons to the standard approach. I have used some of these chapters (with modification) as articles in national magazines and received very favorable comments from across the country.

Exercise methods of my creation are such as: "Time Warp Training, Cumulative Contractions, Positive Stack Progression, Dynamic Symmetry Contractions, Power Partials, Tantric Contractions and the revolutionary "Primordial Principal." Each proven approach is documented by studies with numerous people.

The Primordial Principle is the first accurate method of creating a maximum muscle contraction during the lifting and lowering movement of resistance training. Its use has reduced strength training to only one time per week.

To my knowledge, I was the first person to conduct research and publish the results, comparing the common three workouts (or more) per week, to a format of only two workouts per week. Well received, this two-workout approach is a valuable advance any consumer would greatly benefit from.

The Chapter on: "Potential Injuries Using Nautilus Equipment", to my knowledge the only advice ever printed about the possible injuries produced by misuse or poorly supervised use of Nautilus equipment and other kind of high-tech equipment.

Naturally, since most manufacturers have copied the Nautilus design, those potential injuries are possible on their equipment also.

Most fitness center owner's and instructor's are not aware of the injury potential. Many do not understand that some of the aches and complaints of client's are caused by improper training methods and poorly designed equipment.

Strength Training for Women Only ©

Looking back to 1986 when I wrote the first edition of this book, few if any, books existed speaking to this subject. Now, strength training for women is becoming a popular subject.

Women are finally figuring out that the only quality they lack when compared to men is strength. Once one attains strength, the quality of life improves and if one is involved in sports, personal performance improves.

Guaranteed to improve dramatically a woman's strength and fitness level in a very short time.

Fitness Therapy ©

This is a comprehensive "How to" management and marketing book containing a step by step approach to improve one's image and income in the fitness business and explains how to establish success in the physical therapy field.

Highly personal, it identifies with the state of the present fitness center owner's who are caught in the circle of traditional Business practices, which in my opinion, has reached critical mass.

Many fitness center owners would like to cross over into the therapy market. This book points a way into the medical industry and outlines its potential traps. Following the procedures can produce an astronomical increase in one's business income.

As you know, a typical fitness center earns about $3.21, or less, per client visits. The average therapy clinic earns $72 per visit for the same service—supervised exercise.

When first tested marked to a select group, this book sold at a price of $79.95. Now mass-produced the price is more in line with traditional book prices.

I received many calls about this approach and the name Fitness Therapy. At one time, I was not heavily marketing this book or others.

I authored under the copyright title of the Fitness Therapy name and concept. It went so well, I was scheduled to introduce this concept in Las Vegas at a national trade show, but I canceled due to family reasons.

Naturally, thanks to the cutthroat nature of the fitness business, a competitor was scheduled to speak on my concept and eventually wrote a book of the same name. It is not generally known but, book titles are not protected by the Copyright laws, so anyone, qualified or not, can use the name of any book previously published.

In short, if you are searching for an honest, no punches pulled approach to the fitness, physical therapy, or work rehabilitation issues, and a sane, individualized approach to legitimate fitness training, you can purchase our products expecting and receiving the best knowledge available.

ABOUT THE AUTHOR

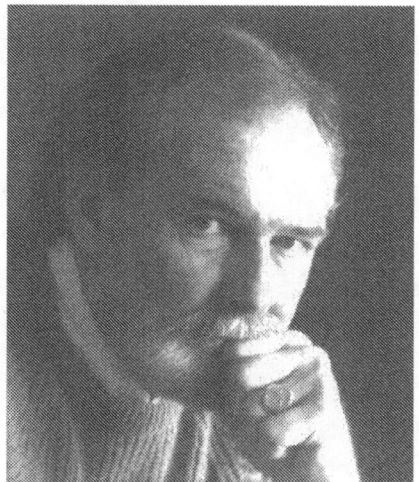

The purpose of this book is to educate and entertain.

Joseph Mullen continues his involvement in fitness, proactive physical therapy, work performance, bodybuilding, and weightlifting. This journey continues for more than five decades.

Initially attracted to exercise to increase his strength and muscle size; he became a title winner (New England's Strongest Man, East Coast Strongest Man, Massachusetts Arm Wrestling Champion); national judge (A.A.U., I.F.B.B) in women and men physique competition and arm wrestling; a featured performer in a traveling strength show; a show promoter, and trainer of many men and women title winners.

He dedicated the years from 1950 to 1970, to training him and others, towards the goals of high-level fitness and sports competition, with the aid of progressive resistance exercise tools.

At the same time, he conducted health and fitness research, attempting to find the most time efficient, cost effective method of developing wellness. The only progressive resistance exercise tools available were barbells, dumbbells, and wall pulleys. High tech exercise tools were not yet invented.

20 years of knowledge and experience, proved valuable, when the health and fitness industry, shook to its roots. Arthur Jones, and his high tech invention, Nautilus exercise equipment emerged.

Joseph understood its potential and the impact high-tech would have on health and fitness training and physical therapy.

Realizing high-tech exercise would spawn a new breed of health and fitness centers, he began his association with Nautilus on the ground, floor opening the first successful Nautilus equipped club in New England in the early 70's.

There was virtually no management or marketing information available to help pioneer the high tech approach to exercise or therapy.

Like many pioneers, Joseph learned through trial and error. While this method proved successful, it was costly and time consuming. Eventually, he created a formula for indoctrination, supervision, education, and motivation of members, which worked miracles. He has owned nine fitness and physical therapy centers.

In 1980, he became a staff member of Nautilus Sports/Medical Industries and The Nautilus Television Network in DeLand, Florida

His duties were wide-ranging and included: producer of television programming; writing for national magazines, including Nautilus Magazine; speaking at National Nautilus Seminars, marketing consulting to fitness professions;, and research.

In 1989, he was appointed Northern California Regional Director, for MedX West and began research into time efficient, cost-effective physical therapy

The Author of this book, writer for national magazines, and numerous appearances on radio and television as a consumer advocate, he is credited with changing the lives of untold numbers of fitness and wellness enthusiasts. He shares his knowledge with you through this book. Use it to your advantage.

He continues his leadership in the fitness and physical therapy professions with his latest books, Life Force Fitness Therapy and Strength Training for Women Only.

For more information about his services, visit his web sites

www.lifeforcefitnesstherapy.com or ww.californiastrengthinstitute.com,
Or, write him at
safe-life@worldnet.att.net.

0-595-28017-X

www.ingramcontent.com/pod-product-compliance
Lightning Source LLC
Chambersburg PA
CBHW061311280526
45784CB00002B/961